Body<u>Instinct</u>

6-Week
TOTAL Transformation Program

By Tari Rose

www.TariRose.com

Copyright 2011

Cover Photos: LynnParks.com
Makeup/Hair: Tatjana Terzic
Interior exercise photos: Aida Gillete

ISBN: 1460966392
ISBN-13: 9781460966396

ACKNOWLEDGEMENTS

To my wonderful family – My husband Jack who has been so patient, supportive and encouraging! My kids - Tommi and Maxim who give me inspiration on a daily basis and could say "no hydrogenated oils" from the age of 3!

A special thank you to my Dad and my many friends who I called on many times in many emails for their opinions and advice! To my Mom for inspiring me by starting her own exercise studio back in the 70"s in our basement and always making sure we ate healthy!

I also want to thank all of my many clients over the years who have touched and inspired me with their successes!

FORWARD

"You are what you eat"…..is only partially true. "You are what you eat…..after 3pm" is the real truth! There is too much emphasis on what we're eating and not enough on when we're eating it. Timing is everything! Discover the proven strategy of eating in sync with your circadian rhythm. Did you know that even timing your exercise properly can burn 10 times more body fat every day and significantly reduce the amount of time you need to exercise??? Based on my 20 years of extensive professional experience in the health & fitness industry "The BodyInstinct Total Transformation Program", is the one truly effective comprehensive nutrition AND fitness program designed to give you all the tools and knowledge you will ever need to create the healthiest most fit body possible. No magic pills, powders or special equipment needed! If you need to lose 5 pounds or 105 pounds BodyInstinct is the way to do it! Teach your body to burn fat for you 24 hours a day! Apply this instinctual way of eating and exercising to keep you and your entire family lean and healthy for life!

In this book you will discover how to:

- Make food, exercise and your body's metabolism work together most efficiently and in sync with your circadian rhythm to give you maximum results!
- Effectively choose **what** you eat and **when** you should eat it to get leaner.

- Erase your fear of food groups like fats and carbohydrates and find out how they can actually help you to lose body-fat when eaten at the right times!
- Exercise smarter to burn the most fat and create the leanest, strongest, healthiest most fit body possible with minimum time invested!
- Start the most effective exercise program you can do or tweak your current exercise program to make it 10 times more effective!
- Shop for healthier foods and products. Learn the hidden secrets behind the labels!
- Naturally increase energy levels!
- Enjoy your favorite foods and still get lean and healthy!
- Make the best choices when eating in restaurants, at parties, traveling or on the run.
- Avoid pesticides, genetic engineering, growth hormones, antibiotics and other   potentially dangerous additives in your food.
- Apply this instinctual way of eating and exercising to keep you and your family lean and healthy for life!

BODYINSTINCT CHAPTER OUTLINE

INTRODUCTION: EATING INSTINCTIVELY AND WHY

CHAPTER ONE - WEEK ONE: GETTING STARTED
- Cardio training - Exercising less but harder is smarter-the truth about cardio & fat burning
- Eating Instinct #1: Unprocessed foods are the key: If you can't read it, don't eat it
- Eating Instinct #2: Eating in sync with your Circadian rhythm
- Eating Instinct #3: Keep The Fire Burning-metabolism & fat
- Eating Instinct #4: Fats: The good, the bad & the ugly
- Eating Instinct #5: Drink water burn fat
- Eating Instinct #6: The importance of Protein
- Eating Instinct #7: Late night eating=more body fat
- BodyInstinct Food Sheets
- BodyInstinct Suggested Shopping list

CHAPTER TWO - WEEK TWO: THE BALL IS ROLLING
- Strength training – Creating a lean strong fat burning body
- Cardio training - The best time to exercise to burn the most fat
- Eating Instinct #8: You are what you eat – after 3:00 pm
- Eating Instinct #9: Alcohol and your health
- Eating Instinct #10: Don't drink your calories

CHAPTER THREE - WEEK THREE: YOUR INSTINCTS KICKING BACK IN!
- Cardio Training – Even *more* time can be on your side
- Eating Instinct #11: Satisfy your sweet tooth without sabotaging your body
- Eating Instinct #12: Sleep your way to a leaner body

INTRODUCTION

EATING INSTINCTIVELY AND WHY

Achieving and maintaining a healthy & fit body has become a national obsession. There are countless diet books, fitness videos, fitness centers, health & fitness "experts" and endless nutrition and fitness information in magazines, in newspapers on TV and on the web. All of this information and opportunity to have a healthier more fit body and yet, according to the Center for Disease Control 68% of Americans are overweight and 34% are obese with those numbers increasing every year. How is that possible???

It's possible because people are being misled and implementing unrealistic nutrition and fitness programs and ideas. You may be one of the millions of Americans who have tried and failed on one of the following categories of diets or nutrition programs:

1. The programs that pick one food group and decide that one particular food group all by itself is the demon behind our weight issues. For years it was fat! Food manufacturers jumped on the opportunity and suddenly there was a "fat free" version of everything. Fat free products took over the shelves. People were literally terrified of fat. Nobody ate fat for 10 years and nobody got any skinnier or healthier. We all ended up with dry skin and more body fat! Now, the new enemy is carbohydrates. Evidently, since fat wasn't the culprit, it must be the carbs! Now everyone is scared to death of bread, rice and pasta. No matter where I go, someone is proclaiming that they no

longer eat carbs because carbs make you fat. Carb free products have now replaced the fat free products on the shelves!!! Yet, with all of these people now avoiding carbohydrates, Americans are still getting fatter! Do you see a pattern here? What's next? Protein?? That's the only food group left to pick on!

2. Next comes the diets or programs that micromanage everything that goes into your mouth by forcing you to buy their prepackaged meals. Ok, so what happens next? Do you continue to buy their food for the rest of your life or do you eventually go back to eating like a normal person in normal situations and gain everything back that you lost?

3. Finally, there are the nutrition "experts" who are too vague and simply suggest we just make healthier choices and that alone will get us where we need to be. Well that just simply doesn't work either. You can easily still get fat on healthy foods depending on when you consume them and how much you consume of them.

The tried and NOT true fitness categories aren't much better:

1. First there are the programs that suggest amounts of exercise that are unrealistically excessive. Who in their right mind wants to exercise 6 days a week for an hour or more like many of these programs suggest? How long do you possibly think you can keep that up? What do you think is going to wear out first, your joints or your motivation? Probably both at the same time.

2. Then there is the opposite end of the spectrum: those magazines, books and videos promoting cute little microscopic workouts that you can do in less than the time it takes to microwave a bag of popcorn and supposedly get a super fit body like the person on the cover! Do you honestly think that person got that way doing quickie workouts? I don't. In fact I *know* they didn't.

Right now in your hands are all the answers you will ever need to create a lean strong healthy body and the means to maintain that body for the rest of your life. No matter who you are or what you may perceive to be your limitations in obtaining a healthy fit body. I am a living example of "if she can do it, anybody can". Think obesity genes are too hard to conquer? Think again. I have a strong family history of obesity. I have watched many family members struggle with obesity and I was concerned from a very young age that my genetic predisposition to obesity would be a challenging obstacle to overcome. Yet I was able to do it quite easily with the BodyInstinct Program. Think your age is making it impossible to achieve the body you want? Think again! I am in my late 40's and I can honestly say that this is the best my body has ever looked and felt. Think having children "wrecks" your body permanently? Think again! I have two children and I had them at age 37 and 40. Did I mention they were both over 9 lbs???

I am not bragging but simply demonstrating to you that if I can do it with:

1. a predisposition to obesity
2. being in my late 40's and
3. having had two children

Then ANYBODY can!!!

BodyInstinct is my life's work as a health and fitness consultant. A journey which really began at the age of 18 when my classical dancing career was cut short after becoming paralyzed from the neck down with Guillian Barre syndrome. I realized the bodies tenacity first hand in the year long rehabilitation that followed in which I had to learn to basically do everything (including walking, writing, feeding myself) all over again. My new-found respect for the human body set me on a new track, one of ultimate health & fitness.

The next 20 years of my life were devoted to acquiring as much knowledge and experience as possible in the fields of fitness and nutrition. Although my education was invaluable, my greatest knowledge came from my hands on experience through the years with my many clients of all different ages, shapes and fitness levels. All with unique issues but all with the same goal: to get the leanest, strongest, healthiest most fit body possible with minimum time invested. It was through this trial and error experimenting with my client's bodies and my own body, that I saw firsthand what worked and what didn't. The most interesting part was that what DID work, worked for everyone!! A lot of what I found went against what the rest of the health and fitness industry was doing at the time but it worked and it was safer and healthier.

So, keep in mind as you start the BodyInstinct Program that no matter what you have tried before that hasn't worked you will now have everything you need to experience great success with minimal effort! Or if you've never tried any fitness or nutrition program before you are in luck! BodyInstinct will be your first *and* last and you won't have to build your own personal library of fitness and nutrition books that don't work.

This program will teach you the way we were intended to eat and the way we would be eating today had we been permitted to follow the natural eating instincts that we were born with. What I do with this program is the opposite of what most nutrition programs do. Most try to teach you a new way of dieting. I am going to teach you a long forgotten way of eating! I am going to take you back to your primary eating instincts to what should be your natural way of eating. After the initial adjustments, you will find that it really is very simple. After all it's your natural born eating instincts back at work. What could be easier than that? You already have everything you need. It's just sitting there waiting to be uncovered! Together we will strip away the conditioning, which has blocked your natural eating instincts. The conditioning I'm talking about is the unnatural eating habits that have been imposed on us by society, our well-meaning families, and just our modern day world in general.

THEY CIRCADIAN RHYTHYM CONNECTION:

Probably the strongest driving force behind our eating instincts is our circadian rhythm. Circadian rhythm is the 24 hour cycle in the biochemical, physiological and behavioral processes of all living things. Our circadian rhythm determines our sleep/wake cycles and our metabolic cycles. Learning to eat in sync with your circadian rhythm instead of against it is going to turn your body into a body fat burner instead of a body fat storer! You are about to find out why _**when**_ you eat is just as important as what you eat!!

HOW IT WORKS:

The program is progressive, meaning you start out making a few small changes in your eating habits the first week and then a few more each week thereafter. Before you know it, you've changed your eating habits completely and it feels perfectly comfortable and natural because it's your body's own instincts kicking back in. Instead of doing an abrupt lifestyle change (which is what most programs do) the BodyInstinct program kind of sneaks up on you. At the end of six weeks you will be noticeably leaner, healthier, and more energetic. At that time, I'll put you on a maintenance program which will continue to produce results for you indefinitely.

NUTRITION & EXERCISE GO HAND IN HAND:

During the course of the next six weeks, I will also design your cardiovascular/resistance exercise program for you. If you are already doing some type of cardiovascular/resistance activity, I will teach you how to tweak it in ways that will burn 10 times more fat and tone more muscle. If you aren't currently exercising I will encourage you to begin a program that will be very effective, convenient & comfortable for you. You will learn how to produce maximum results with minimum time invested!

GETTING STARTED!!!

I know you are excited to get started! It's very important to keep in mind before we do get started with this program that our main goal is to lose body fat and conserve lean muscle. Lean muscle sets our resting metabolic rate so, the more lean muscle you have the more calories you burn just sitting on the couch or driving your car or sitting at your desk! It is NOT humanly possibly to lose more than 1-2 pounds of *pure body fat* a week. So, if you have dieted before and lost more than 2 pounds a week, then you certainly sabotaged your metabolism by losing lean muscle. This is why the diets that claim huge instant weight loss like 5 – 10 pounds in your first week NEVER work! The minute you lose more than 2 pounds a week you will lower your resting metabolic rate and your fat burning potential and when you go off the diet (which is inevitable with diets so restrictive) you will most likely gain all of the weight back (if not more) and the next time you try to get the fat off, it will be even harder because you now have less muscle tissue and therefore a lower resting metabolism. This kind of instant gratification thinking and super restrictive dieting ultimately drags your metabolism down lower and lower each time. No wonder it seems like it gets harder and harder to lose weight! It does if you continue to do this to your body.

That being said, it is important for you to know that the BodyInstinct program is NOT some quick fix lose a lot now and gain it all back later program. BodyInstinct was designed to give you a permanent body fat loss of 1-2 pounds per week for as long as you want to keep losing! This program takes 6 weeks to fully implement but is intended to be used for a lifetime! You will never have to feel that you are dieting again. You will only be making changes that allow your natural instincts to take back over your body and give you new eating and thinking habits. The ideas presented to you in this program can be implemented any-where, anytime. Any restaurant, vacation, family get together, party, or special occasion can still be enjoyed while using the pro-gram. The BodyInstinct Program will forever change the way you think about food and fitness. Change your thoughts, change your body, change your life!!!

ONE LAST THING.....

This book contains one chapter for each week of the six week program. Each chapter begins with a list of Fitness Guidelines and Eating Instincts for that week followed by an explanation intended to give you as much knowledge as possible as to how that particular Fitness Guideline or Eating Instinct will move you closer to a leaner, stronger, healthier body. Knowledge is power! The more you know about how and why something is good for you, the more likely you are to follow it and stick with it! Each week we will build upon what we have already learned and imple-mented with new Fitness Guidelines and Eating Instincts. The new guidelines and instincts for that week will be printed in bold letters so you can differentiate. I encourage you to resist the temptation to read ahead and instead focus on what you are sup-posed to be changing and implementing for the particular week you are in. Live in the moment and enjoy the journey!

BODYINSTINCT "6 WEEK TOTAL TRANSFORMATION PROGRAM"

WEEK 1
FITNESS GUIDELINES:

__Cardio program:__ Three 20-minute cardio workouts a week done very intensely in an interval fashion. 4 minutes at or above your 75% range and the 5th minute at full blast then repeat this 4 times total to complete 20 minutes. Warm up and cool down do not count towards the 20 minutes. A heart rate monitor is highly recommended to make sure you are burning fat most efficiently. (To find your 75% range: 220 – your age x 75%)

NUTRITION PROGRAM EATING INSTINCTS:

- __Eating Instinct #1:__ Eat unprocessed foods whenever possible (food in its natural state). Your diet should consist mainly of lean high quality protein, fruits & vegetables.
- __Eating Instinct #2:__ Be a daytime eater. Always eat breakfast, make lunch your main meal, and think of dinner as a small light meal, consisting of lean protein and vegetables.
- __Eating Instinct #3:__ NEVER let more than 3 hours go by without food. Eat several small meals instead of 2-3 big ones or supplement 3 regular meals with healthy unprocessed snacks such as fruit, veggies or nuts in between.
- __Eating Instinct #4:__ Avoid most saturated fat and __all__ hydrogenated oils (trans fats). The fat in your diet should be coming mostly from nuts, seeds, olives, and avocados. (oils should be used sparingly and should be cold or

1

expeller pressed) Remove all products with hydrogenated or partially hydrogenated oils from your home.

- **<u>Eating Instinct #5:</u>** Drink at least 48 oz. (6 cups) of water every day.
- **<u>Eating Instinct #6:</u>** Make sure you are getting lean high quality protein at least 3 times a day.
- **<u>Eating Instinct #7:</u>** Avoid eating after 7:00 pm or 12 hours after regular wake up time.

CHAPTER ONE:

GETTING STARTED

FITNESS GUIDELINES:

Exercising less but harder is smarter – the truth about cardio & fat burning

<u>Cardio program</u>: **Three 20-minute cardio workouts a week done very intensely in an interval fashion. 4 minutes at or above your 75% range and the 5th minute at full blast then repeat this 4 times total to complete 20 minutes. Warm up and cool down do not count towards the 20 minutes. A heart rate monitor is highly recommended to make sure you are burning fat most efficiently. (To find your 75% range: 220 – your age x 75%)**

For the past 20 years or so, most fitness experts have stated that if you want to lose fat you must exercise longer. I myself bought into that train of thought and passed it onto my clients in my early years as a fitness trainer. The most popular recommendations were (and still are) to do 30 – 60 minutes of cardiovascular training 5 to 6 days a week. What I found out from that experience was, not only were the individuals following that advice getting burned out mentally and physically, over time they actually gained weight! My "in your face" example of how too much cardio is not a good thing was when I took a position running a health club on the beach in Fort Lauderdale. For most of the 5 years I was there, I would open the doors every morning at 6:00 am and each morning the same 10 people would wander in the door. All of them would go right over to the cardio area where a wide variety of cardio machines were available for them to choose from. Elipticals, treadmills, stationary bikes, you name it, it was there! For at least 30-60 minutes each morning, these ten individuals would mindlessly run walk, or bike like hamsters on a wheel. They would then leave soaking ringing wet with sweat looking as though they had really done something. Now, you would think (as they did I'm sure) after that much consistent effort, the results would be fantastic! Yet, year after year of watching this faithful morning ritual of these well intended folks, the sad truth was, NONE of them ever lost any weight, in fact, about half actually gained weight during those 5 years!!! Ten different people of different genders, ages, and body types doing different types of cardio every day and not one of them achieved any promising results!! That is downright sad and discouraging! If you've ever belonged to a fitness center for any length of time, I'm sure you've observed the same phenomenon yourself. Or maybe when you go outside every morning you see that same guy running down your street again. That same guy whose body has not changed one iota in the 3 years he's been running by your house every day. Seems like a lot of effort for little or no results!

Why? You ask, would individuals doing that much exercise not lose and possibly actually gain weight?

Well, it's a combination of these three things:

1. Research shows and I can tell you first hand that when you are doing 30 minutes or more of cardio a day most days of the week, you increase your appetite. The body resists change and that much activity causes your body to signal you to eat more to make up for all the calories you

4

are burning. Years ago before I created the BodyInstinct program, I was personally doing 30 minutes or more of cardio every day and I was ALWAYS hungry!!!

2. When you are doing that much cardiovascular activity your body begins to burn not only fat but lean muscle which in turn sabotages your resting metabolic rate. As I described in the introduction, you want to hold onto or increase your muscle tissue at all costs because that is what determines how many calories you burn when your body is at rest, which is most of the day. Even though individuals doing a lot of cardio for a long period of time may be burning significant calories while exercising, some of those calories are muscles being burned up for fuel ultimately killing your metabolism for the rest of the day!

3. The common misconception that "I am doing so much cardio that I should be able to eat as much as I want". Well the reality is YOU CAN ALWAYS OUT EAT YOUR WORKOUT!!! Example: if you spend an entire hour on the treadmill or doing any other method of cardio, the absolute most you are going to burn is about 350 to 400 calories. One small smoothie later at your favorite juice bar and your right back where you started. If it were possible to work out enough to eat absolutely as much as you wanted then there wouldn't be any overweight fitness instructors. Every time I speak at or attend a fitness convention, my observations are that more than half of fitness instructors are overfat. Some of these individuals are teaching (and doing) over 10 classes a week yet they still are overfat. Lesson learned: never attempt to use your cardio as a tool to burn the calories you are consuming.

As I mentioned earlier two other big reasons for cutting back on the cardio is physical and mental burnout. Doing excessive amounts of cardio eventually almost always leads to joint, ligament and tendon problems otherwise known as overuse injuries. Just about every person that came through that fitness center door who engaged in excessive cardio developed some type of painful overuse injury. Case in point, when I personally was a victim of excessive cardio I found myself each morning wrapping both ankles and one knee with athletic support bandages just to get out the door to go for a run! Then I would come back and ice all 3 joints as well to avoid pain. One day I stepped back and looked at myself and just shook my head! This was anything BUT health & fitness!!

The last reason for avoiding excessive cardio is mental burnout. How long do you think you can keep up doing 30-60 minutes of cardio 6 days a week, 52 weeks a year? One year, 5 years, 10 years? It's mentally exhausting just thinking about it! It's important to know that most people give up on an exercise program because it's too overwhelming mentally and physically to think that you have to keep up with that much exercise for the rest of your life.

INTENSITY DETERMINES FREQUENCY AND DURATION:

Hopefully, by now, you're convinced that excessive cardio is not the path to a leaner stronger body. Instead, we are going to *increase* the *intensity* of your cardio workout which will in turn *decrease* your need for *frequency* and *duration*. In other words, you will work harder but for shorter periods of time and for fewer workouts per week. Not only will this type of training decrease mental burnout, physical burnout and overuse injuries but most important it will get you leaner faster!!! Doesn't that sound great??? Less is more!! Now that I have your attention, let's see exactly how this new type of cardio training will work for you by examining the principles of cardio training stated in week one:

TYPES OF CARDIO EXERCISE:

Question: What type of cardio is the best type of cardio to do??? Biking? Walking? Running? Treadmill? Elliptical machine? Or something else?

Answer: The best type of cardio for you is what you like to do best! (or what you dislike the least) The reason is simple: the more you like what you are doing the more likely you are to do it. You may already be doing your favorite type of cardio and want to stick with that, or maybe you want to try something else. You may not be doing any cardio training at the moment or may have never done any at all. In any case, make a choice and if it doesn't suit you then choose again. Have a short attention span? Then mix it up! You can walk or run one day and bike the next! Don't like hot or cold weather? Then exercise inside in a controlled environment. Don't like gyms or feeling like a hamster on a wheel? Then take it outside! The point is: IT'S ALL GOOD!!!!

HOW MUCH CARDIO?

Wouldn't it be great if someone told you that 20 minutes of cardiovascular exercise done 3 times a week could get you leaner faster than anything else? Well, I'm here to tell you it's true! If you want to create a leaner stronger healthier body than all you need to do as far as your cardiovascular or fat burning exercise is concerned is 20 minutes 3 times a week!!!! That sounds so much better than 30-60 minutes a day for 6 days a week! Done properly, in an <u>interval training</u> fashion, that 20 minutes is going to move fat off of your body quicker and more permanently than those marathon workouts! Maximum results with minimum time invested!

WHAT IS INTERVAL TRAINING?

Although I have been preaching and practicing interval training for years with my clients and myself, Interval training is an up and coming style of cardiovascular/fat burning training that is just now catching on with other fitness experts. The latest research is overwhelming as it points to study after study that show fat burning ability increased by 39% or more in individuals who switched to interval training. Studies aside, I can produce example after example of my own clients who came to me at the end of their rope after years and years of unproductive cardio who, now are leaner, healthier, more energetic and happier doing my interval style of cardio training. They are doing less and achieving more.

Traditional cardio exercise uses slow twitch muscle fibers (or endurance muscle fibers) almost exclusively. Interval training is traditional cardio exercise activity with short quick bursts of energy thrown in. These quick intense bursts of energy known as "intervals" recruit the fast twitch muscle fibers (speed and power) of your body along with the slow twitch fibers (endurance). The use of these fast twitch fibers create more muscle tone and increase your body's ability to burn fat. In other words, your body recognizes that you are now doing a more intense workout and realizes that it must not only save all muscle tissue you have but actually increase your muscle tone and burn significantly more fat as fuel. Wow! How great is that??? Let's do it:

GETTING THE ABSOLUTE MOST OUT OF YOUR WORKOUT!!

Before you even think about starting your new cardio program, it is an absolute must that you purchase or use a heart rate monitor! I am adamant about this with my clients and even myself. You may think you are pretty good at estimating what your heart rate is at any given time (perceived exertion) or even checking your own pulse. In my experience both are very inaccurate.

Perceived exertion is inaccurate because your body responds to exercise differently most every day. Your heart rate can change due to a small difference in your sleep patterns or sleep duration, your stress level, what you ate the day before, or even the weather. When I am doing my cardio exercise I always try to guess what my heart rate is before I look down at my monitor and I am incorrect by 10 beats or more 50% of the time. So, as a trained professional, if I am no good at it, you probably aren't either. Taking your pulse is also a poor way to determine your heart rate because you have to slow down or stop just to be able to take it, which, obviously, changes your heart rate. Also, during interval training, your heart rate changes so much and so often that it is almost impossible to complete an effective workout without a monitor.

No need to spend a lot of money here. A bottom of the line heart rate monitor from a good company like Polar Target Heart Rate Monitors will be a small expense and last you possibly a lifetime. You don't need all the bells and whistles some heart rate monitors offer. Just a watch that displays your heart rate with a band that goes around your chest. I personally use the cheapest Polar Target Heart Rate monitor. It serves as a watch, displays my heart rate, beeps if I go too low out of my range, and lets me know how long I've been exercising. Best of all, its user friendly. Just one button!!! So, get your heart rate monitor and leave no room for error!!

DETERMINING YOUR HEART RATE RANGE:

Although, you will be adding quick intense bursts of exercise intermittently during your cardio, you will also be using a higher sustained heart rate in between those interval bursts than what you may be used to or may have been told to use before. For the intense fat burning muscle building purposes of your new cardio workout, you will be working at or above your 75% heart rate in between those interval bursts. The formula for finding your 75% heart rate is simple:

220 – your age X 75% = your 75% heart rate

Example: if you are 45 years old:

220 – 45 = 175 x 75% = 131 (75% heart rate)

The number you come up with using the above formula will be the lowest your heart rate should go during your 20 minute exercise session. In other words, your heart rate should be at or above your 75% heart rate the whole time. We are not going to concern ourselves with the highest your heart rate should go because, in interval training, your heart rate can go very high for a brief period of time. In fact, during your speed/power intervals, you should work up to going as hard as you possibly can during that minute.

YOUR NEW FAT BURNING FORMULA:

You now know that you are only responsible for 3 – 20 minute cardio workouts a week done in an interval fashion. Let's break one of those 20 minute workouts down and examine it a little closer:

20 minute cardio formula: 4 minutes at or above your 75% range and the 5th minute at full blast then repeat this 4 times total to complete 20 minutes.

1. First of all, warm up and cool down DO NOT count towards your 20 minutes. The amount of warm up and cool down a person needs is very individual. A minute might be enough for some while others might need a little longer to wake up their body or to calm it back down.

Like your heart rate, your warm up and cool down needs may change from day to day. Use your instincts here and take the time that you need to warm up enough to be able to get into your 20 minutes at your 75% heart rate or above and keep moving slowly to cool down at the end of your 20 minutes until your breath becomes normal again. It is also important to remember to warm up and cool down "sport specific" which means use whatever type of exercise you are doing as both your warm up and cool down. Just do it a little slower and easier. (e.g. if you are going to fast walk as your cardio exercise, then just warm up and cool down by walking slower.) I would also highly discourage you from stretching before your cardio exercise. Stretching a cold tight muscle is ineffective and can even lead to injury. It is much smarter and healthier to wait until after your workout when your muscles are warm and more flexible to stretch if you'd like.

2. Once you are warmed up and ready to go you should start your 20 minute workout by getting up to or above your 75% heart rate as quickly as possible. Exercise for the first 4 minutes at or above that 75% mark and then do the 5th minute working up to "full blast" or as hard as you can go. Remember that "full blast" is a relative term. It may mean just faster walking for a more de-conditioned person and may be a full out sprint for someone who is more fit. As your fitness level increases so will the intensity of your "full blast" interval. Another point to remember is increasing your speed isn't the only way to up your heart rate for the one minute intervals. You can also increase your resistance. For instance, if you are working out on the treadmill, you can choose to increase the speed *or* the elevation of the machine (which increases the resistance) or a little of both to get your "full blast' interval minute in. If you are walking outside, a hill or some jumping jacks

will increase your resistance without making it necessary to increase your speed. So, either speed or resistance or a combination of both will increase your heart rate for the one minute interval every 5th minute. These 5 minute sets each consisting of 4 minutes at or above your 75% heart rate and the 5th minute working up to "full blast" should be repeated 4 times total to complete your 20 minutes.

This 20 minute BodyInstinct style cardio workout should be done 3 times a week. No more no less. If you are tempted to do longer workouts or more workouts, because you think you will reach your goals quicker, go back and read the section on excessive cardio again and let yourself be talked out of it. If you want to increase something then increase your intensity, NOT your duration or frequency!

FLEXIBILITY HELPS KEEP YOU ON TRACK:

It Does NOT matter what days of the week you do your three workouts. Splitting it up on Mondays, Wednesdays, and Fridays, has no advantage whatsoever over doing it three days in a row such as Friday Saturday and Sunday. If you are the type of person who likes to "get it over with" you can do it Monday, Tuesday, and Wednesday and be done with it for the week. Or if you like to create more balance then split it up throughout the week. All that is important to remember here is to DO your three 20 minute workouts and DO them in the BodyInstinct cardio formula!

a note on strength/resistance training: If you are currently doing some type of strength/resistance training (e.g. weight training, Pilates, toning classes) let it go just for this week and concentrate on your new method of doing cardio. Don't worry you won't back slide in just one week and actually it will do your body good. If you currently aren't doing any strength training then you are good for now! We'll discuss strength training next week!

WEEK ONE EATING INSTINCTS:

*<u>Eating Instinct #1</u>: Unprocessed foods are the key!!!! If you can't read it don't eat it!!

Eat unprocessed foods whenever possible (food in its natural state). Your diet should consist mainly of lean high quality protein, fruits & vegetables.

Eating unprocessed foods sounds like a very simple common sense approach to a healthier diet. Yet, most Americans consume over 75% of their calories from heavily processed foods. What's wrong with processed foods anyway? I could write a whole book just on this subject. In a nutshell:

Food processing generally lowers the nutritional value of foods. Processed foods tend to include food additives, such as artificial flavors, artificial colors, fillers, preservatives and texturizers, which may have little, or no nutritive value, or are just downright unhealthy. Some preservatives added or created during processing such as nitrates, nitrites or sulphites have been known to cause adverse health effects. Processed foods often contain high levels of sugar, corn syrup, or white flour. The high number of calories in processed foods with no nutritional value are referred to as "empty calories". These empty calories literally have nothing to offer except increased body fat and possibly health risks.

Take a box of crackers, bars, or chips out of your cabinets or off of the shelf in the grocery store and read the ingredients. Do you even know what half of that stuff is? Can you even pronounce it? Yet, most still eat it! A good rule of thumb to follow is: "if you can't read it, don't eat it! Or "if you can't identify, don't try" Also, ingredients are listed in the order of content percentage. In other words, the food you are about to eat is composed primarily of the first three ingredients in the ingredients list. If one of the first three ingredients is either sugar or corn syrup, you probably want to put that back too.

Don't be fooled by processed foods claiming to be "health foods". There are absolutely no guidelines set down by the FDA to limit the use of these words. It is just a marketing term with usually no scientific basis for the claim. Even those so called granola or protein "health" bars are heavily processed foods. You would be far better off carrying around an apple or banana in your purse or briefcase.

One of my favorite "in your face" examples of how unhealthy processed foods are comes from a popular family resort on the East coast. My family and I happened to be visiting there and we had just walked out of one of the restaurants at the resort and were taking a walk outside on the porch. The porch overlooked a lake occupied by many different types of waterfowl and animals. It was there I spotted this sign posted on the wall:

Please – Do Not Feed Food Items From The Restaurants To The Ducks, Birds, Fish, Turtles or Alligators. Processed Food Of This Nature Will Be Harmful To Them. THANK YOU FOR STAYING WITH US

Obviously the resort was much more concerned about the health of their animals than their guests! I see the same thing all the time with people everywhere I go. They will hand their child a processed snack of some sort and when the child goes to share it with the family pet, the parent will run over and intervene telling the child "don't feed that to the dog, it will make him sick". How ironic is that??? What are you telling your child? It's ok for you but Fido deserves better healthier food???

Enough focusing on what we shouldn't eat, let's turn it around and focus positively on what we should eat. Unprocessed foods or foods in their natural state (also known as "whole" foods) give us the most bang for our buck! Foods like whole fruits and vegetables, lean cuts of protein, eggs, beans, nuts and seeds. These foods are highest in nutrient value and are also stocked full of the vitamins, antioxidants, and amino acids our bodies need to thrive and function at their best.

Processed foods are all around us. In vending machines, convenience stores, grocery stores, fast food restaurants and even upscale expensive restaurants. The good news is that all of the places I just mentioned also offer unprocessed or minimally processed whole food choices as well. It's up to you as the consumer to make the best choice. Here's a little help:

Vending machine
Instead of chips or crackers choose a bag of peanuts

Convenience store
Instead of a granola bar or candy bar choose a small bag of pistachios/banana

Grocery store
Instead of boxed and bagged food in the aisles shop the perimeters of the grocery for fresh veggies, fruits & lean protein.

Next time you walk up to that vending machine, choose the bag of peanuts instead of the granola bar, at the convenience store, grab that banana or a small bag of pistachios. In the grocery store, avoid the isles as much as possible and shop the perimeters of the store where most of the unprocessed healthy foods are usually stocked. Skip the protein bar and throw some raisins and nuts in your bag.

Fast food restaurants even offer choices such as chili, salads, grilled chicken breast, sliced apples. Also, when spending time and money at a pricier restaurant stick to the grilled fish, chicken or lean steak with lots of yummy vegetables, beans or salads.

Eating primarily unprocessed or minimally processed foods will increase your energy, help you to get and stay lean and make you look and feel so much healthier, vibrant and younger! Starting right now, take most or all of the heavily processed foods out of your diet and see for yourself!

*<u>Eating Instinct #2:</u> *Eating in sync with your circadian rhythm!* **Be a daytime eater.**

Always eat breakfast, make lunch your main meal, and think of dinner as a small light meal, consisting of lean protein and vegetables.

Our Circadian rhythm establishes our sleep/wake cycles and metabolic processes in a 24 hour cycle. It is endogenous to the human body which means it comes from within and persists in the absence of cues such as light, persists in any temperature and will adjust itself to match the time zone that you are currently in. In fact the syndrome we call "jet-lag" is actually the body's circadian rhythm adjusting to the new time zone. If you have ever experienced jet-lag you have seen firsthand how disrupting your circadian rhythm has a strong influence on your body. It can and does produce feelings of disorientation, fatigue, insomnia, loss of concentration, loss of energy, digestive problems, headaches and general malaise. It is proof positive that being out of sync with your circadian rhythm is not a good thing.

In the same respect, *eating* out of sync with your circadian rhythm has a strong influence on your body as well with an unde-sired effect: major fat storage. Your circadian rhythm controls

16

your metabolism. Your metabolism starts out strong and is at its highest point early in the morning when you wake up and it slowly goes downhill all day until it's at its lowest point at the end of the day before bed. Just as your metabolism starts out strong and ends slow your eating should follow that pattern too.

The old adage I used to hear my grandmother say is so true:

"Eat breakfast like a king, lunch like a prince and dinner like a pauper". They really knew something back then and we should learn from it. Instead, we as a society have completely flipped the entire adage: most eat little or no breakfast, then choose a small meal or a light salad for lunch and then by the time they arrive home in the late afternoon or evening, they are starving and eat a big dinner ingesting the majority of their calories late in the day when they are most likely to end up being stored as fat.

It makes so much more sense to "frontload" your calories or eat most of your calories earlier in the day when they are more likely to be burned up as energy. Driven by our circadian rhythm your metabolism is movin' and groovin' during the day. Even if you have a desk job, your metabolism is still higher and burning more calories during the day than it is later in the afternoon and evening. We need to learn to get back to our instinctual way of eating for our energy needs. Since our energy needs are greater in the first half of the day, that's when we should be consuming the most calories.

If you are one of those individuals eating a small breakfast or completely skipping breakfast altogether I am sure I am not the first one to tell you that this is not a good idea. There are many studies that show and have shown for years that individuals who skip breakfast are much more likely to become obese and to develop heart disease. These individuals also have higher and earlier rates of mortality. Eating lunch as your first meal of the day sabotages your metabolism and your blood sugar causing increased hunger later in the day and more deposition of body fat, especially in the abdomen.

Question: "I'm simply not hungry in the morning. Should I force myself to eat?"

Answer: YES! You have trained your body not to be hungry in the morning by eating too many calories the evening before. In fact, one of the obvious signs of eating too much late in the day is not waking up hungry. A healthy fit body wakes up hungry. To accomplish a reversal in your eating habits to get back to your instinctual way of eating you need to do 3 things:

1. Cut back on your dinner portions. Immediately begin to make dinner a small light meal consisting mostly of lean high quality protein and vegetables. Stop eating completely after dinner.
2. Start eating something for breakfast! Even if you have to start out small with a bite or two of banana or a handful of cheerios you can eventually increase to a meal.
3. Stop skimping on lunch! If you love having a salad for lunch great, but, eat some protein like fish or chicken and some fibrous starches with it like whole grain bread, beans, brown rice or whole grain pasta.

All 3 of these changes work best when done together. Each one helps you to accomplish the other two. Start by eating a good breakfast or at least start getting your feet wet with a little something in the morning. Then at lunch eat a more satisfying meal and then at dinner it will be easier to eat a smaller meal. The next morning when you wake up you should be hungrier than you are used to and able to eat a bigger breakfast and so on and so on. Within one week you should be able to totally reverse a lifetime of self-defeating eating habits. When you start to wake up hungry every morning, you will know you have done it!

__Eating Instinct #3:__ *Keep the fire burning-metabolism and fat.*

NEVER let more than 3 hours go by without food. Eat several small meals instead of 2-3 big ones or supplement 3 regular meals with healthy unprocessed snacks such as fruit, veggies or nuts in between.

Instinctually we are natural born grazers. A baby is born when it is hungry it eats, when it is satisfied it stops. As soon as it becomes hungry again it will eat again and soon as it is satisfied again it stops. It naturally knows when and how much it needs to eat. This process of eating only when hungry and stopping when satiated would continue throughout the child's entire life if it weren't for one thing...............adult human intervention.

How many times have you seen a mother try to entice a baby to nurse long after the baby really has no more interest in eating because she wants to finish the bottle? Or on the flip side, a mother delays the request of the infant for food because of inconvenience. Just about every baby book advocates trying to get your child on a set feeding schedule to make it easier and more convenient for the parents. It's this type of intervention that begins the process of stripping away a child's natural instincts to better conform him or her into a more convenient and accepted schedule. The price of this convenience is being out of order with your natural eating instincts.

Soon the infant becomes a small child. Studies have shown that a small child if left to their own devices would graze all day long without ever eating a so called "meal". That's because at this point in their development (up until the age of 4 or 5) their instincts are still very strong and still resisting conforming to 3 regular meals a day.

Unfortunately, sooner or later, they are required to conform to a society where we eat breakfast, lunch and dinner. The child learns that he won't necessarily get to eat whenever he chooses so, when he does get the opportunity to eat he will have the tendency to eat as much as he *can* instead of how much he actually *wants*. Familiar phrases like "no snacking in between meals or you'll spoil your dinner" and "finish everything on your plate" also encourage the child to ignore their natural hunger instincts. Delaying a child food when they are hungry or forcing a child to sit down and eat when they are not hungry strips the child of their natural instincts and begins the problem of consuming too many calories at one time and eating past satiety.

Now, that child is you, an adult who most likely overeats to some extent at breakfast lunch and dinner to take in enough food to get you to the next meal which may be 5 or more hours away. Because society has made it almost impossible to remain a natural grazer people generally stuff themselves 2 or three times a day taking in way more calories at one time than their bodies can possibly burn, so the additional calories get stored as body fat.

An even bigger problem with eating only 3 meals a day is the effect it has on your metabolism. Taking in too many calories at one sitting and then not eating again until many hours later, ultimately slows your metabolism down so that it's even less equipped to deal with the calories at your next meal and encourages your body to store even more fat. When the body goes without food for 3 or more hours, it becomes "worried" and goes into starvation mode conserving energy expenditure and calories. Simply, It's your body saying "hey, It's been a long time since I've been fed and I don't know when he/she is going to feed me again so, I'm just going to stop burning as many calories until I'm sure I'm getting more food". Your body's metabolism then slows down considerably, burning less and less fat and calories with each minute that passes after 3 hours. It's kind of like a fire in a fire place. It's important once you get that fire started to consistently add wood to the fire so it doesn't go out because once it does go out it's difficult to get it started up again. It's the same with your metabolism. Obviously it doesn't stop or "go out" like the fire but, it can slow down to almost a crawl.

One of the foundations of the BodyInstinct program is to get your body's metabolism working *for* you instead of against you. One of the ways this can be accomplished is to make sure that your body never goes more than 3 hours without food. Grazing is definitely the way to go to keep our metabolism revved up and calorie intake spread out more evenly throughout the day however, most people are so far removed from their natural grazing instincts that it is going to take some manipulating initially to get them to kick back in. This is why it's not a good idea, as many diets suggest, to just graze all day long eating whenever you want because with your instincts suppressed, even with healthy foods, you can graze your way right into obesity. Think about it: cows are grazers. So, instead of "eating all over the place" with no sign of your instincts to tell you when enough is enough, you are going to think: "controlled grazing".

One method of accomplishing "controlled grazing" is having 5 or 6 small meals each day. Although, some programs will suggest you do this and it does work, it is not practical or realistic when it comes to everyday life. If you like the idea of preparing 5 or 6 small meals in containers neatly stacked up in your fridge for the day or carrying them around with you in a cooler, than knock yourself out. Not only does this take a tremendous amount of forethought and preparation every day, but there is a huge social aspect you're missing here. What happens when your co-workers want to take you out to lunch? Do you refuse the desired social invitation in fear of the prepackaged meal in the mini fridge not being eaten? How about when it's time to dive into your last Tupperware container and a loved one eagerly suggests dinner at your favorite local eatery? Do you decline or do you go but feel all "freaked out" because this was not in the food plan for the day??

Another way that will work just as well and is much more doable is eating a sensible breakfast, lunch and dinner and supplementing those 3 regular meals with healthy unprocessed snacks such as fruit, veggies or nuts in between. One snack in between breakfast and lunch and another in between lunch and dinner will do the trick. This type of eating is more like grazing, the way we were intended to eat and would be eating today had we been allowed to follow our natural instincts.

What exactly constitutes a "snack" do you ask? An optimal snack would be one whole fruit or 1 cup of fruit pieces along with some type of nuts or seeds. Your nut/seed serving is very individual as it is one handful of nuts/seeds per day. Your hand works perfectly as a measuring device for your body size: Small frame, small handful, large frame, larger handful. In other words, choose your favorite nut/seed or nut/seed mixture and get your hand in there and grab as many as you can with one hand (if any fall out they're not yours). Put that handful of nuts/seeds in a plastic Ziploc or other container and that is your own personal nut/seed allotment for the day. You can split that baggie full of nuts/seeds into two servings if you choose, eating half with a piece of fruit in between breakfast and lunch and the other half in between lunch and dinner with more fruit. You can also take your fruit and nut servings and slowly snack on them all day in between meals.

What type of fruits and nuts are best? All fruits and nuts are full of different yet wonderful nutrients, vitamins, minerals and antioxidants offering tremendous health benefits. Eating a variety of fruits and nuts is your best bet to achieving a healthy body. It makes me crazy when the media reports on a study of one particular fruit or nut and suggests eating that particular fruit or nut every day to achieve optimum health. It's funny how people just get all crazy and run with that stuff. Case in point: On a recent visit to my uncle's house I opened his freezer to get some ice and was assaulted by bags and bags of frozen blueberries falling out at me. When I inquired why his freezer was full of nothing but ice and blueberries he told me he had heard on the news that blueberries were the best fruit for you and to eat them every day.

He was literally afraid of running out of this "miracle fruit". I explained to him that yes, blueberries do have a lot to offer a body but, so do oranges, apples, bananas, etc. and he wouldn't want to be missing out on the amazing health benefits and nutrients other fruits have to offer.

A common misconception is that you need a substantial snack or meal every 3 hours to keep that metabolism going. Actually, just the *introduction* of food does the trick. As long as your body recognizes that you are putting in calories, even in super small amounts, it will not crash your metabolism. *Example:* if you are in a business meeting and it's coming up on your three hour mark and you know you can't eat your full snack just yet, you can throw a nut or two from your snack into your mouth to hold you over and to keep your metabolism burning until you can get to the rest of your snack.

To drive home the point of how important it is to keep your metabolism burning, I often tell clients that ultimately if you are approaching that 3 hour mark and the only food available is m&ms, it would be better in the long run for your body's metabolism and your fat burning to eat a few of the m&ms then to eat nothing. Remember, I'm trying to make a point with this statement. Don't take this one comment and run with it or before you know it this will be known as the m&m diet!

It's also important to remember that it's not necessary to eat *exactly* every 3 hours, there might be anywhere from 1½ to 3 hours in between meals and snacks depending on your circumstances that day and what time you happen to be eating your meals. 3 hours is just the absolute longest you should ever go in between eating.

Question: "I'm not really hungry for a snack in between meals, should I still eat it?"

Answer: Yes! Remember you have conditioned yourself not to require food in between meals and suppressed your natural grazing instincts so we must initially do some manipulating to get them back. Eating the snack will also start to require you to need less food at your 3 main meals.

After just one week of watching the clock and making sure you are not letting any more than 3 hours go by without food, your body's natural instincts will automatically kick back in and your body will "ask" for food when it needs it and you will find that you are no longer able to go more than 2 or 3 hours without food. It's amazing how quickly your instincts kick back in on this one!

*<u>Eating Instinct #4:</u> *Fats! The good, the bad, and the ugly!*

Avoid most saturated fat and all hydrogenated oils (trans fats). The fat in your diet should be coming mostly from nuts, seeds, olives, and avocados. (oils should be used sparingly and should be cold or expeller pressed) Remove all products with hydrogenated or partially hydrogenated oils from your home.

It wasn't long ago when fat was considered the enemy. It was blamed for everything from heart disease to obesity. It didn't even really matter what kind of fat. Fat was bad and that was that. Every food product suddenly had a fat free version and people were literally terrified of eating fat. After over a decade of a nation eating little or no fat, no one became any thinner, and in fact, more people than ever were becoming overfat and obese. Now we know much more about fat. Not all fats are bad for you, some fat is necessary, and some fats are better than others.

Fat is necessary in the body to provide energy, to aid in the absorption of fat soluble vitamins F, A, D, E, and K, to surround and protect vital organs, and to insulate the nervous system. In addition, fats enhance the taste of food and create a longer lasting feeling of fullness after a meal.

If none of that convinced you it's important to eat fat, then this will: *you need fat to burn fat.* If you are trying to get fat off of your body, you must be taking in some fat to accomplish this. If you are starving your body of fat it will react by conserving the fat on your body in fear of limited fat resources. Your body will simply refuse to burn your fat as a preferred fuel source until it is assured you are going to be consistently taking in fat on a daily basis.

Your types of fat choices are very important:

POLYUNSATURATED AND MONOUNSATURATED: (The Good) mostly found in nuts and seeds, these fats are optimal and necessary fats for your body. They primarily come from plant sources such as vegetables, nuts, olives and seeds. Unsaturated fats are usually liquid at room temperature. These are the preferred fats but still should not be consumed in excess. For example, some people have taken the fact that olive oil is beneficial for you as a license to saturate everything they eat with it and then wonder why they're gaining weight! Oils are a processed food. It takes one whole quart of olives to make just one teaspoon of olive oil! Would you ever sit down and eat one quart of olives at a sitting? No, you probably wouldn't, but if you did you would get all of the fiber and pulp in the olives that nature intended to be consumed along with the oil in the olives. You can see how unnatural it is to consume olive oil or any other oil in large amounts. It would be much better for you if you actually ate the olives, nuts, or seeds instead of the oil extracted from them. Just the way nature intended. As mentioned previously, nuts and seeds can be a great snack and useful tool for grazing.

Use oils sparingly for cooking or dressings and make sure your oils are cold or expeller pressed. (It will be printed right on the front of the label) Oils extracted through heat or chemical methods have most of their nutrients destroyed in the process. It is also important to remember to keep all nuts, nut butters, seeds and oils in the fridge after opening. Oils and foods containing oils can become rancid at room temperature. Rancid oils produce free radicals and have been found to be carcinogenic and a health hazard to the body. Peanut butter can actually form dangerous aflotoxins if left at room temperature. So if you're not going to blow through that bag of nuts or bottle of olive oil in a week or less, stick it in the fridge after you crack the seal or open the bag.

Some fats that are getting a lot of attention lately due to their tremendous health benefits are Omega-3s. Omega-3 fatty acids are a form of polyunsaturated fat that the body derives from food. Omega-3s (and omega-6s) are known as essential fatty acids (EFAs) because they are important for good health. These different types of acids can be obtained in foods such as cold-water fish including tuna, salmon, and mackerel. Other important omega 3 fatty acids are found in dark green leafy vegetables, walnuts, chia seeds and flaxseed.

According to the American Heart Association: Omega-3 fatty acids have been found to be beneficial for the heart. Positive effects include anti-inflammatory and anti-blood clotting actions, lowering cholesterol and triglyceride levels, and reducing blood pressure. These fatty acids may also reduce the risks and symptoms for other disorders including diabetes, stroke, rheumatoid arthritis, asthma, inflammatory bowel disease, ulcerative colitis, some cancers, and mental decline.

Along with all the positive health information we are finding out about Omega-3s come recommendations to consume fish oils and flax oils. Bottled and encapsulated omega 3 oils are available everywhere. I highly suggest you avoid these bottled oils and capsules and eat the fish and flax instead! Mainly for 3 reasons:

1. Bottled fish oils and flax oils are considered supplements and are not currently regulated by the FDA. Who knows if what they say is in them is actually present in the bottle. No government agency is really checking on them. Studies have been done by independent companies such as Consumer Labs who randomly pull these products off of store shelves and test them for content. Many times these

oil supplements contain little or none of the beneficial oils they are claiming to offer. Several have been found to contain more coconut oil or palm oil than the beneficial omega 3's.

2. Omega 3's are intended (just like the oil in the olives) to be consumed with the other nutrients that come in the fish or the flax. It is in combination with these other nutrients that Omega 3's can work their magic in the body best.

3. When a nutrient, vitamin or mineral becomes the "in" thing, we have a tendency in this country to go into excess. Fear based advertising and articles feed on our health insecurities and make us believe that we need whatever it is they're pushing and we need it in massive quantities. They want us to believe we couldn't possibly consume enough of the stuff so supplement, supplement, supplement! If a little is good then a lot must be better! Food manufacturers jump on the hype bandwagon and suddenly start fortifying foods with omega 3's that have no business containing omega 3's. At this moment there are cereals, breads, milk and even orange juice fortified with omega 3's! The problem with fortifying foods with any nutrient or vitamin is then you run the risk of too much of a good thing. Case in point: In 1998 the FDA began requiring enriched grains to be fortified with folic acid when it was discovered the vitamin was instrumental in preventing birth defects. All Breads, crackers, cereal and many other foods suddenly had an extra helping of folic acid. Add that to the increase in folic acid in vitamins and many Americans without even being aware of it, were taking in double or triple the amounts of the recommended daily allowance of folic acid. Then in 2007, after nine years of folic acid fortification in our food, studies began to show an increase in colon cancer blamed on too much folic acid in our diets! Imagine that! Actually the studies have

shown that small amounts of folic acid *decrease* cancer risk yet large amounts *increase* cancer risk. The theory "if a little is good then a lot must be better" is not a good motto to eat by. My concern is (and yours should be too) that fortifying foods with whatever the "in" nutrient, vitamin or mineral is at the moment may have long term repercussions that we will not be aware of until it's too late since the studies of adverse effects usually don't show anything until many years later.

SATURATED: (The Bad???) Saturated fats come primarily from animal sources such as meat and dairy. Saturated fat is usually solid at room temperature. This fat was the "bad" fat for many years and still leaves many running scared. In reality, saturated fat is not evil and your body is well equipped to deal with moderate amounts in the diet. Remember that we are omnivores and our bodies are designed to eat, digest and utilize saturated fat. There is saturated fat in breast milk and it is an integral part in an infant's development. My suggestion is to limit your intake of saturated fat keeping it at or below 10% of your food intake.

Saturated fat is often associated with high cholesterol. Some foods such as eggs which contain saturated fat and are high in cholesterol were exiled for years from the American diet. Now evidence shows that cholesterol found in foods does not transfer into cholesterol in our bodies. Your body manufactures its own cholesterol. Some of that cholesterol is good cholesterol (HDL – think "H" for high, which is what you want it to be) and some is dangerous (LDL – think "L" for low, which is what you want it to be). Be careful with placing too much importance on what your total cholesterol level is. You may have been told that a cholesterol level of 200 or lower is optimal and an overall cholesterol over 240 is high. However, the single number your doctor may give you conceals more than it reveals. It's the ratio of HDL to LDL within that number that is important. In fact, your HDL should be as high as possible! It's scary to think that some doctors still to this day are giving only one number to patients to gauge their cholesterol. Recently a mom of one of the little girls on my 7 year olds soccer team came to me in a panic. She said that on a routine visit to the pediatrician, her 7 year olds cholesterol had come back high on a blood test and was told that she should get some nutritional advice to lower it. Through further investigation, I learned that the mother had not been told what her child's LDL and HDL levels were only that the overall number was high. I advised her to have another test done through an independent lab and request both HDL and LDL levels. It turned out that the child's HDL levels were high raising her overall number yet, the LDL levels were low. The child was perfectly healthy with great independent cholesterol levels.

Since we've learned that just because a particular food is high in cholesterol it really doesn't mean much to your own personal cholesterol levels, what *does* encourage your body to manufacture its own cholesterol? Well, saturated fat does in the sense that too much saturated fat in the diet encourages the production of your LDL cholesterol (the bad one). Doctors and institutions like the American Heart Association have been telling us for years to avoid saturated fat blaming it for obesity and heart disease. However, since we are omnivores by nature and were designed to be able to consume animal meats and fats it seems odd that what nature designed our bodies to consume would eventually do us in. To add to this train of thought there is more and more evidence every day that the real culprit of high cholesterol, high blood pressure and heart disease and the most dangerous fat of all is the man made fat:

HYDROGENATED OILS aka TRANS FATS: (The Ugly) Hydrogenation is an industrial process in which normally healthy polyunsaturated and monounsaturated oils are converted into unhealthy more solid forms of fat. Food manufacturers do this to improve the shelf life of their products. (I guess they're not too concerned about our "shelf life".) Partially hydrogenated oils are commonly found in processed foods like commercially baked products such as cookies, cakes and crackers, and even in bread. They are also used as cooking oils for frying in many restaurants.

Trans fats were first introduced to grocery stores in 1911 in the form of Crisco. Since then product after product has been infused with these lethal fats. Did you know that most peanut butters and margarines are full of trans fats?? For decades we were told to stop eating butter and eat margarine to be healthier when in fact, margarines are nothing but huge tubs of trans fats!!! We would have been much better off eating butter!! Think how much artery clogging trans fats we took in *just* in the form of margarine in the last 30 years!

The national academy of science (NAS), the American Heart Association (AHA), The Food and drug administration (FDA) and the department of Health and Human Services (HHS) have all determined that there is NO safe level of trans fats in a healthy diet! These recommendations are based on the facts that trans fatty acids are non essential and provide no known benefit to the human body and even more important are extremely detrimental to the human body due to the fact that *any* incremental increase in trans fat intake increases the risk of coronary heart disease.

Although over consumption of saturated fats are known to raise our LDL (bad) cholesterol, *any* consumption of Trans fats can cause a significant increase in LDL (bad) cholesterol *and* significant lowering of HDL (good) cholesterol! A double whammy! They also make the arteries more rigid; cause major clogging of arteries; cause insulin resistance; cause or contribute to type 2 diabetes; and cause or contribute to other serious health problems.

Considering the overwhelming evidence now would be a good time to go through your kitchen and throw away anything and everything containing trans fats. Don't be fooled by products claiming in big bold letters on the front of the package that they contain "no trans fats". The FDA has a little deal with the devil. Although the FDA has required all products to now claim trans fats in the nutritional facts box on all labels, they are allowing products containing less then ½ a gram of trans fats *per serving* to claim they contain zero trans fats!!! That is just ridiculous! Remember that a company can define their own serving size so many products have not changed their trans fat content only their serving size! Let's say that a cracker company once had a serving size of eight crackers, which contained .8 grams of trans fats. They would have to claim that on their label. Or they could just change their serving size to 4 crackers bringing the trans fat content down to .4 grams which in accordance with FDA regulations could be claimed as no trans fats!!! This is just unbelievable to me! If that box contains 20 total servings of crackers, then that box contains 8 grams of trans fats yet, can claim it has none!!! Realistically, you could consume 10 or more grams of trans fats per day eating only products that claim they contain "no trans fats". So, how do you know if the products you are buying contain trans fats? Read the ingredients list. If anywhere in the list of ingredients you see the words "shortening", "partially hydrogenated", or "hydrogenated" put it back! It contains trans fats.

How about restaurants??? Many restaurants cook with trans fats or serve products containing trans fats. Don't think that just because you are eating in some high-end restaurant there aren't any trans fats in your food. By the time you leave some fast food joints or gourmet eateries, you could have easily consumed well over 10 grams of trans fats! How do you know if your favorite restaurants use and serve trans fats? You can ask or most chain restaurants have websites listing their nutritional information and food ingredients.

You may have read or seen in the news that New York City banned all partially hydrogenated frying oils in all restaurants as of July 1st 2007. After some initial whining, the change went smoothly. My question is if the removal of trans fats from all frying oils in New York City was accomplished fairly easily, why can't all cities follow suit or better yet, the entire country?

You may not be able to control what restaurants are doing but, you have complete control of what is served in your home and stocked in your fridge and cabinets. Remove it, get rid of it, don't feed it to the dog or give it away, throw it in the trash. Make sure you read all labels on all foods. Remember, no food is exempt from the possibility of containing trans fats. Check your peanut butter, creamers, cereals, baked goods (even those from bakeries), chips, popcorn, dry seasoning packets, etc.. Refuse to buy any products containing ugly trans fats. Do yourself and your family a BIG favor!!!

Excess dietary fat, especially trans fat, is a major cause of overweight and obesity and a contributor to heart disease, hypertension, diabetes, some cancers, and other illnesses.

Most experts suggest that no more than 30% of daily calories should come from fat, with little coming from saturated and none from trans fats. So, there you have it, the good, the bad, and the ugly of fats. Try incorporating your new awareness into your dietary selections.

*<u>Eating Instinct #5:</u> *Drink water burn fat!!!*

Drink at least 48 oz. (6 cups) of water every day

We all have heard for our entire lives that water is good for you! You may or may not know that it can help you beat a fever, improve your complexion, relieve constipation, build muscle, drain a stuffy nose, fight a stomach ache, improve your mood and help you to burn fat. What??? Help you to burn fat? Yes! Take for example, identical twins. Both eating the exact same foods and exercising for the same intensity, duration and frequency. The only difference is twin A is consuming healthy amounts of water and twin B is not consuming enough water. At the end of 6 weeks, twin A (the water drinker) would have less body fat than twin B! Most health books and fitness magazine articles recommend an adequate water intake to help you burn more fat yet, have you ever been told exactly *how* that works? I have always believed that knowledge is power and the more you know about how something works, the more apt you are to implement it. That being said, here is a simplified explanation of how water helps your body to burn fat:

Your liver and your kidneys are the major detoxifiers of your body. The kidneys have jobs that are specific to them and the liver has jobs specific to it. However, there are some jobs that are shared by the kidneys and the liver. It is important to know that the liver in addition to being a major detoxifier, is the one and only organ that metabolizes your stored body fat. In other words, in order for *any* of your body fat to be burned up as fuel it has to be metabolized by your liver. Keeping all of this in mind, your kidneys need plenty of water to function properly and do their jobs (specific and shared) 100%. If you do not give your kidneys the water they need to do all of their jobs properly, they will concentrate on the jobs only they can perform and slack off on the jobs they share with the liver.

The liver then has to pick up the slack and do most or all of the shared jobs by itself. Since the liver is suddenly overloaded, something has to give. Can you guess what that will be? Well, detoxifying the body is a higher priority than burning fat so, yep, you've got it: fat burning! If you are not adequately hydrating yourself you are setting your body up to store fat!

We are going to start this week by consuming at least 6 cups (48 oz.) of water every day. Don't assume that you drink lots of water and you must be consuming at least that amount. Just to make a point, measure out the required amount with either the water bottles or glasses and cups you use and be sure to consume that amount every day. If you haven't by the end of the day then you should drink the remaining water before you go to bed and it might not be fun running to the john all night.

You may or may not already be a big water drinker. Some of my clients have no problem with this part, others are more challenged. If you find it challenging to drink 6 cups of water a day, I can give you a little hint: drink a big glass first thing in the morning (when your body needs it the most) and down a glass before every meal. Your stomach is empty or close to it at these times so it's easier to get the water in. Also, drinking a glass of water before each meal will decrease your calorie intake at that meal because if your body is at all deficient in water when you sit down to eat, it will cause you to eat more in search of water in your food. One more great reason to drink your water!

No other liquids containing water (e.g. tea, sodas, juices) count towards your required water intake. Cutting back on these will help you to take in more water as well. As your water intake increases, you will burn more fat and discover where every restroom in your city is!

*<u>Eating Instinct #6:</u> *The importance of protein!*

Make sure you are getting lean high quality protein at least 3 times a day.

Every cell in the human body contains protein. It is a major part of the skin, muscles, organs, and glands. Protein is a repair and recovery food. You need protein in your diet to help your body repair cells and make new ones. If you are going to exercise and expect your body to respond favorably you need to make sure you are getting protein at least 3 times a day.

There seldom seems to be an issue with my male clients taking in enough protein. Most males are higher protein eaters instinctively. Their quality of protein might not always be so good (e.g. sausage, pepperoni, etc.) but, at least they are drawn more towards protein foods. My female clients on the other hand are almost always lacking in protein intake when they come to me. You may have heard some conflicting advice on protein intake over the years. Depending on who you talk to or what you read, there are many different protein recommendations out there. Some are too general recommending the same amount of protein intake for men and women from too wide an age range of 19-70 without taking into account body size, activity level and muscularity. Other recommendations are too specific and suggest an exact amount of protein per pound of body weight. Although those take into account body size, they still don't address activity level or body composition not to mention they are annoying since counting of any kind (calories, protein grams, carbs, etc.) is impractical and just a huge pain in the butt.

The more muscle you have the more protein you need to support that muscle. Protein is so important because one of our main objectives here is to increase muscle to raise our resting metabolism. If you are doing everything you need exercise wise to increase your muscle thus increasing your resting metabolism, but you fail to get enough protein, your muscles will not have the building blocks they need to repair and recover from your workouts and you will not see the results you desire.

How then, you ask, do you ensure you are getting enough protein? Very simply, make sure that you see some form of lean high quality protein on your plate at breakfast lunch and dinner. What exactly does "lean high quality" mean? "Lean" is obvious, although you need not be terrified of saturated fat, as mentioned in our fats conversation, you don't want to be eating tons of the stuff. "High quality" on the other hand refers to how efficiently certain proteins are used by the body. Proteins are grouped as compete and incomplete. Complete proteins contain all 9 essential amino acids. Complete proteins which are the most efficient protein for the body are mostly animal products such as meat, fish, poultry, and eggs. Soy is the only plant protein that contains all 9 essential amino acids and is therefore a complete protein. One or two decks of cards are the perfect size if you need to be more specific. You can refer to the protein sheet at the end of this chapter for suggestions on protein sources. Also, your handful of nuts divided into two or more snacks throughout the day will supply your body with another source of protein intake throughout the day.

Be careful with individuals, books, and articles suggesting high amounts of protein in the form of protein shakes, bars and supplements. Remember that too much of a good thing almost always turns bad!

*<u>Eating Instinct #7</u>: *Late night eating = more body fat!*

Avoid eating after 7:00 pm or 12 hours after regular wake up time.

What time to you get up in the morning *most days* of the week? 6, 7, or 8am maybe? Take the time you wake up most days of the week (Monday thru Friday) and replace the AM with a PM and that is the latest you should be eating on a regular basis. In other words, 12 hours after your regular wake up time should be your eating cut off point. I've had some clients try to wheel and deal with me on this one: "well I get up at 6 but I don't eat breakfast until 8". Doesn't matter what time you start *eating* it matters what time you *wake up*! As we learned in eating instinct #2 your body works on a metabolic clock controlled by your circadian rhythm that pretty much shuts down (or tremendously slows down) your metabolism 12 hours after you wake up turning much of or all of what you eat after that 12 hour mark into fat. Since this world has turned people into breakfast skippers, light lunch eaters, and heavy late night eaters, this eating instinct may be one of the most challenging to apply. However, it is also one of the most reward-ing if followed! The good results of not eating after 7:00 pm or 12 hours after your regular wake up time come fast and furious.

For most people this pretty much means an earlier dinner and no snacking after dinner. The beautiful part about this and the entire BodyInstinct program is that you don't need to do this 100% of the time to see results. If you like later dinners on the weekends or have a business dinner a couple of nights a week but can still manage to pull off 4 or 5 nights a week with an earlier dinner then you will still do great! Change your thinking from "uhhhhhhhh, I have a birthday dinner to go too late Friday night and a late business dinner to go to on Thursday, which is really going to mess me up" to "Hey, 5 nights this week I was able to stop eating in my 12 hour time frame! Great!" Also, what you can do when confronted with eating late is remember to follow the "eat dinner like a pauper" eating instinct! If you've eaten your breakfast, lunch and snacks correctly, that shouldn't be a problem. If you are eating out, you should know that almost every meal served in a restaurant in this country is at least double what you should be eating for dinner. Remedy this by immediately halving everything on your plate when it arrives and taking half your dinner home with you in a doggie bag. Other options are to order an appetizer instead of a dinner or focus on lean protein and vegetables.

Cutting off your eating after an earlier dinner is an amazing way to help you stay lean for the rest of your life. Instinctively it's what we should be doing. Think about the word "breakfast". It says it all. Waking up in the morning and eating is "breaking a fast". 12 hours after our regular wake up time should be the start of that fast. Remember, a healthy body wakes up hungry!

Additional commentary on week one:
There you have it! Your first week and you're up and running! A few notes to get you on your way:

- Remember to resist the temptation to look ahead to week 2 and instead live in the moment putting all your efforts into the week one exercise and eating instincts! Week 2 will be here before you know it!

- Familiarize yourself with the food source pages at the end of this chapter. They are broken down into the food groups: protein, starchy carbs, fats, vegetables, and fruits.

- There is a "suggested" shopping list as well. This is to mainly give you ideas of new foods that you might want to incorporate into your kitchen. In no way am I suggesting you go out and buy all this stuff. There are things on the food sheets and shopping list that don't necessarily appeal to me but they may appeal to you and vice versa! These lists are a compilation of my food suggestions and food suggestions brought to me by clients over the years! There are also items that are directed more towards vegetarians if you happen to be one.

- Doing the BodyInstinct program is a life changing experience. You will never look at food and fitness the same again. I highly suggest you journal your food and exercise experience. Any small notebook will do or keep track of food intake on your computer or in a blog. One of the most important reasons to journal, even if you are not going to share it, is to have this information for yourself. Keep it simple, just jotting down time you ate and what you ate. Quantities are not necessary to list unless you want to. Also, write down when you exercise. In the future if you get off track or start to ignore your instincts, you can always look back at your journal and see exactly how you were eating and exercising when you were really looking and feeling good!

- One last thing: The BodyInstinct program has many ideas, concepts and tweaks to implement into your life. If you are not doing everything I throw at you 100% every day, that's ok!!! This is not a program you are "on" or "off"; you are just doing it to the best of your ability on a day to day basis. Think of it more as a percentage. Obviously, if you are following the program 100% every day you are going to get maximum results but, if you can do the program 80% or more, you will still see good results! If you missed the boat on a couple instincts today but were able to implement many others than that is great! I like to tell my clients, you determine your own success. The more you do it, the more success you will have!!

PROTEIN

Serving size is 1 or 2 decks of cards unless otherwise noted

LEAN RED MEAT – When possible choose leaner cuts such as eye of round, top round, round tip, & top sirloin. USDA select grade has the lowest amount of fat. Trim all visible fat before cooking. Maverick Ranch or Coleman are healthier brands due to the absence of steroids or antibiotics. Many grocery store chains now offer their brand of organic or steroid free meats. Check with your local grocer.

SKINLESS CHICKEN BREAST - When available, choose free range or a brand with minimal additives and processing such as Perdue, Murray's or Bell Evans. Costco and most grocery chains now carry organic chicken at better prices than health food stores.

CHICKEN NUGGETS – Bell & Evans brand, or both Tyson and Perdue make Dino nuggets for kids. Or make your own!

SKINLESS TURKEY BREAST - Available sliced or as a whole breast for baking.

GROUND TURKEY BREAST - Make sure it is ground turkey *BREAST*. Regular ground turkey has more fat than lean ground beef. Turkey Store is a good name brand.

LOWFAT COTTAGE CHEESE *½ cup*- Can be mixed with fruit, spaghetti sauce, nuts, veggies, cinnamon, or just by itself. Perfect for your morning protein. Organic is a better choice.

LOWFAT TURKEY SAUSAGE - Cook with green peppers and onions for a great dinner. Turkey Store is a good brand.

LOWFAT BEEF OR TURKEY DOGS *1-* Make sure they are nitrate and nitrite free. No artificial anything. Applegate Farms or Coleman All Natural are good brands for beef hotdogs.

LEAN DELI MEATS - brands with no nitrates, no nitrites and no preservatives or artificial ingredients such as Boars Head All Natural are a better choice.

TOFU - Throw in just about anything or marinate and grill.

ALL FISH - Any fish grilled, poached, broiled, steamed, or baked.

ALL SHELLFISH - any shellfish prepared same as above. Be cautious of raw shellfish.

LEAN PORK - Choose a leaner cut such as tenderloin, 95% lean ham, boneless sirloin chops. Whenever possible choose brands produced without antibiotics or additives. USDA select grade has the lowest amount of fat. Maverick Ranch is a good brand or your local grocery chains organic brand is good too.

LOWFAT CHEESE *1 deck of cards-* Choose minimally processed and use sparingly. There are many different brands. Read labels and stay away from artificial anything and ingredients you don't recognize. Organic is a better choice.

BUFFALO – Good choice for lean red meat. Antibiotic and steroid free; buffalo are still raised in roaming herds.

BOCA BURGERS, DR. PRAEGER BURGERS, VEGGIE BURGERS & GARDEN BURGERS - Excellent tasting and a great source of soy protein.

MORNINGSTAR FARMS PATTIES - Another good lowfat soy product. Great for breakfast!

BEANS/PEAS *½ cup (tennis ball)* - any and all varieties including but not limited to: black beans, pinto beans, chick peas, garbanzo beans, kidney beans, navy beans, northern beans, lentils, pintos, black-eyed peas, hummus, refried beans without lard.

NUTLETTES - (texturized vegetable protein) *Use ¼ cup* added to cereal for your morning protein. Can also be added to oatmeal or other hot cereals. Available at some health food stores and online at www.dixiediner.com

SMART DOGS *1* - Made from soy.

EGGS – (Up to two whole eggs a day). Scrambled, omelet, hardboiled, soft boiled, or poached.

EGG WHITES - *2* -4 per serving

LEAN BACON – *2 -4 slices* No nitrites or nitrates. Cook in microwave between paper towels until crispy to get rid of most of the fat. Welshire Farms and Maverick Ranch are good brands.

SEITAN - Wheat gluten protein. A meatloaf type consistency.

CANNED TUNA - Chunk Albacore is the best choice. Read labels and stay away from anything artificial or unrecognizable. Also, Starkist makes seasoned tuna fillets in foil pouches in the canned tuna section.

CANNED CHICKEN BREAST - Make sure it is *BREAST* with nothing strange or artificial added. Swanson is a good brand.

OSTRICH - A very lean high quality protein available in most health food stores. More like red meat

ARNOLD DOUBLE PROTEIN BREAD – can be used occasionally for your protein at breakfast lunch or snack. Not dinner.

FAGE YOGURT   (**lowfat**) - *½ *cup* high protein yogurt with no growth hormones. Much better choice than protein powders for shakes.

STARCHY CARBS

Starchy carbs are energy food and should be eaten early during the day when you expend the most energy. Look for minimally processed products with no artificial colors, flavors, or preservatives. Make the best choices whenever possible.

serving size is a baseball size (1 cup) cooked unless otherwise noted

CEREALS - *1 cup dry* preferably whole grain such as Nabisco Shredded Wheat & Bran, Kashi, regular Cheerios or Kix. Rule of thumb when choosing cereals: Fiber content should be over 3 grams per serving and sugar content should be less than 5 grams per serving.

OATMEAL – *½ cup dry* preferably Quaker Old Fashioned oatmeal, organic whole oats, steel cut oats, wheat oats or rye oats, Kashi instant packets, Quaker organic instant packets, Quaker Simple Harvest Packets.

CREAM OF WHEAT - *1/3 cup dry* preferably whole wheat

CREAM OF RICE - *1/3 cup dry* Preferably brown rice

RICE - preferably brown

POTATOES - any and all varieties with skin on

PASTA - preferably whole grain such as whole wheat or blends such as Barilla or Ronzoni

BREAD - *1 or 2 slices* preferably whole grain. Arnold, Pepperidge Farm or Natures Own are good brands.

TORTILLAS (wraps) - *1 preferably whole grain flour or 2 corn. Flat Out or Tortilla Factory whole grain tortillas are good brands.

SWEET SNACKS - cakes, cookies, muffins, frozen yogurt, candies etc.

WHOLE GRAIN FLOURS - including but not limited to: buckwheat, barley, bulgur, durum, whole wheat, spelt, oat. King Arthur is the best whole wheat flour I have found.

SUGAR - *should be used sparingly as an accent*

BAGELS - *½ or 1 whole bagel scooped, or 1 whole mini bagel or 1 whole bagel thin* preferably whole grain

LOWFAT MILK - *should be used as an accent only and be organic or hormone free*

YOGURT – *1 cup should be organic or hormone free*

SOY MILK - *should be used as an accent only* "Silk" is a good tasting brand.

RICE MILK - *should be used as an accent only*

RICE CAKES - *2 whole grain

PANCAKES - *1-2 whole wheat or buckwheat are best no more than 6 inches in diameter*

BAKED or NATURAL CORN CHIPS - *10 chips* Guiltless Gourmet, Tostitos, Garden of Eatin'

VEGETABLES

Whole fresh vegetables are always your first choice. Look for fresh, local and in season or organic. They can be cooked, steamed, grilled, baked or eaten raw. Frozen veggies are your next best choice followed by canned veggies with no added sugar or preservatives. Any and all vegetables are acceptable, including, but not limited too, the following:

serving size – 1 cup cooked or 2 cups raw

ASPARAGUS
ARUGULA
BEETS
BOK CHOY
BROCCOLI
CABBAGE
CARROTS
CAULIFLOWER
COLLARD GREENS
CORN
EGGPLANT
KALE
MUSHROOMS - any and all varieties
PEPPERS - any and all varieties
BRUSSEL SPROUTS
CELERY
CUCUMBERS
LETTUCE - any and all varieties
LEAFY GREENS
ONIONS
RADISHES
SNOW PEAS
SPINACH
SPROUTS - any and all varieties

SQUASH - any and all varieties
ZUCHINI
ARTICHOKES
CORN
TOMATOES
STRING BEANS
GARLIC
POPCORN – *3 cups* preferably air popped (once a week treat)

FRUITS

Whole fruits are always your best bet. Not fruit juice. Canned and bottled fruit pieces are a second choice but should NOT contain added sugar or fruit juice. Dried fruits are ok but should NOT contain added sugar, fruit juice concentrate, or preservatives. Just fruit! Any and all fruits are acceptable including, but not limited to, the following list:

serving size is 1 whole fruit or 1 cup of fruit pieces

APPLES - Any and all varieties including *all natural* apple sauce.
BANANAS
APRICOTS
BERRIES - Any and all varieties including: blueberries, strawberries, blackberries, rasberries, & gooseberries
GRAPES - Any and all varieties including: seedless, globes, concord, black, red & green
PAPAYA
PINEAPPLE
PLUMS
PEARS - Any and all varieties
CHERRIES
GRAPEFRUIT
KIWI
LEMONS
LIMES
MANGO
CANTALOUPE
MELONS - Any and all varieties including watermelon & honeydew
NECTARINE
ORANGES
TANGERINES
PEACHES

PLANTAINS
POMEGRANATE
STARFRUIT
RAISINS OR OTHER DRIED FRUIT (1 HANDFULL OR 1½ OZ BOX)

FATS

Avoid most saturated fat and ALL hydrogenated or partially hydrogenated oils (trans fats)! The fat in your diet should be coming from mostly nuts, seed, olives and avocados. NOT oils. Oils are processed foods. It would be much better for you if you actually ate the whole olives, nuts and seeds instead of the oil extracted from them. Just the way nature intended. If you must use oils, use expeller/cold pressed and use them sparingly. Stay away from added oils and preservatives. Remember to store any oils, nuts or seeds in the refrigerator after opening the container to avoid oil rancidity. Any and all nuts, seeds, and olives are acceptable including, but not limited to, the following:

serving size is 1 handful per day unless otherwise noted

ALMONDS
BRAZIL NUTS
SOY NUTS
CHESTNUTS
CHIA SEEDS
MACADAMIA NUTS
PECANS
WALNUTS
CASHEWS
PIGNOLA
PISTACHIOS
PEANUTS
POPPY SEEDS
FLAX SEEDS - *1 tbsp* -Grind fresh seeds in coffee grinder and sprinkle 1 tblsp. on cereal or on almost anything (a great source of omega 3 fatty acids). You can also buy flax seeds already ground (flax meal).
SUNFLOWER SEEDS
PUMPKIN SEEDS

COCONUT
SESAME SEEDS
AVOCADOS
OLIVES
ANY NATURAL NUT BUTTERS (PEANUT BUTTER, ALMOND BUTTER, ETC)- *1 tblsp.* Should see a natural oil separation and there should be no extra ingredients. Skippy All Natural and Jiff All Natural are ok too.

BODYINSTINCT SUGGESTED SHOPPING LIST

*NUTLETTES (crunchy soy protein) - added to cereal for morning protein available at www.dixiediner.com

FRESH FRUITS AND VEGETABLES (lots and lots!)

SOY MILK - SILK is a good choice

LOWFAT (NOT FAT FREE) MILK- organic or hormone free

OLD FASHIONED OATMEAL (Quaker)

QUAKER ORGANIC OATMEAL PACKETS

QUAKER SIMPLE HARVEST OATMEAL PACKETS

ALL NUTS AND SEEDS (no added preservatives)

GROUND TURKEY *BREAST*

MARATHON HIGH PROTEIN BREAD or JOGGING BREAD www.GermanBreadHaus.com

ARNOLD DOUBLE PROTEIN BREAD OR PEPPERIDGE FARM SOFT 100% WHOLE WHEAT

*BUFFALO MEAT

LOWFAT ORGANIC COTTAGE CHEESE

NATURAL PEANUT BUTTER (with oil separation) or Skippy OR Jiff All Natural

WHOLE GRAIN PANCAKE MIX AND FLOURS (e.g. Aunt Jemima Whole Wheat)

BAKED CORN CHIPS (Frito Lay, Tostitos and Guiltless Gourmet)

HUMMUS (there is a great brand in most deli sections called Sabra)

SALSA

CORN TORILLAS

WHOLE GRAIN PASTA or blend such as Ronzoni, Healthy Harvest or Barilla

WHOLE GRAIN CEREAL (grams of fiber should be 3 or over, sugar should be 5 or under, e.g. Cheerios, Grape Nuts)

ORGANIC OR HORMONE FREE LEAN BEEF (Maverick Ranch or Coleman are great brands)

LEAN PORK

CHICKEN BREAST Perdue is a good brand but you will avoid antibiotics with organic

EGGS (organic if possible)

BEANS DRY OR CANNED (all types)

BRAGG LIQUID AMINOS (wonderful sauce for veggies, meat, or just about anything, made from soy)

NATURAL LOW SUGAR SAUCES

DRY SPICES

LOWFAT ORGANIC OR HORMONE FREE CHEESE (Cracker Barrel 2% is Hormone free and good!)

SOY, SALMON OR TURKEY DOGS

WHOLE GRAIN BREAD and ROLLS (with NO hydrogenated oils) Arnold, Nature's Own and Pepperidge Farms are good brands

WHOLE GRAIN BAGELS (e.g. Pepperidge Farm whole wheat or Thomas whole wheat mini bagels or Thomas whole wheat bagel thins)

BROWN WHOLE GRAIN RICE

TOFU (if you dare!)

FLAX SEED (whole flaxseeds must be ground in coffee grinder before eating) OR FLAX MEAL

AVO CLASSIC GUACAMOLE (In most deli refrigerator sections)

STARKIST TUNA OR SALMON FILLETS (In foil pouches in canned tuna section)

PAUL NEWMAN MICROWAVE POPCORN

TORTILLA FACTORY TORTILLAS

FLAT OUT TORTILLAS

MAVERICK RANCH, APPLEGATE FARMS, WELSHIRE FARMS OR COLEMAN ALL NATURAL BACON

APPLEGATE FARMS or COLEMAN ALL NATURAL hotdogs

FAGE, OIKOS OR CHOBANI yogurt 2%

BIG SKY BREAD granola

VITA TOPS 100 CALORIE MUFFIN TOPS (In the freezer section) NOT the sugar free

AMY'S BURRITOS

BODYINSTINCT 6 WEEK TOTAL TRANSFORMATION PROGRAM

To Buy or Not to Buy..................Organic?

Does it pay to buy organic? On average, organic food costs 50 –100% more than conventional. Sounds substantial, but then so is growing research that shows pesticides are more prevalent in our food and our bodies than previously thought

The Environmental Protection Agency states: Laboratory studies show that pesticides can cause health problems, such as birth defects, nerve damage, cancer, and other effects that might occur over a long period of time. These effects depend on how toxic the pesticide is and how much of it is consumed. Some pesticides also pose <u>unique health risks to children</u>.

So, do you buy all organic some organic or no organic? Here's a little list for you to take to the grocery store the next time you go. It's called the "dirty dozen": foods you should buy organic as often as possible because they are the most heavily laden with pesticides. This list is the result of over 100,000 studies by the USDA and is updated yearly yet pretty much remains the same. All the fruits and vegetables were washed before testing just as you would wash them in your home but you should keep in mind that pesticide residue is not just on the *outside* of fruits and vegetables making it easy to wash or peel off. Many of the pesticides sprayed on fruits and vegetables are washed down into the soil by rain and irrigation and sucked up through the roots of the plant and end up *inside* the fruit or vegetable.

THE DIRTY DOZEN:

1. celery
2. peaches
3. strawberries
4. apples
5. blueberries
6. nectarines
7. bell peppers
8. spinach
9. kale
10. cherries
11. potatoes
12. imported grapes

Why are some fruits and vegetables more heavily laden with pesticides than others? Some fruits and vegetables have more aggressive pests than others and need to be sprayed with stronger pesticides, multiple pesticides, or need to be sprayed more often.

Unless price is no object, the trace amounts of pesticides found on other fruits and vegetables grown in the United States doesn't really justify paying more however, fruits and vegetables imported from other countries may be another issue. Although many pesticides are banned for use in the US, they are still *manufactured* here and then *exported* to other countries! Other countries then use these dangerous pesticides on their crops and can sell their fruits and vegetables back to us! The Foundation for the Advancements in Science and education reports that over 65 million pounds of US banned or severely restricted pesticides are shipped abroad each year and that the US is importing an increasing amount of fresh fruits and vegetables each year.

The organic label also ensures there are no antibiotics, hormones, genetic modification, and irradiation. So if these are concerns to you then you may want to stick with organic.

Baby food is super important to be buying organic. As I mentioned, pesticides pose unique health risks to children. According the Environmental Protection Agency: Children are at a greater risk for some pesticides for a number of reasons. Children's internal organs are still developing and maturing and their enzymatic, metabolic, and immune systems may provide less natural protection than those of an adult. There are "critical periods" in human development when exposure to a toxin can permanently alter the way an individual's biological system operates.

Other foods you should consider buying organic include meat, poultry, eggs and dairy to avoid hormones and or antibiotics.

I know for many the price of organic produce, meats and dairy can be a deterrent. I am here to tell you I can understand yet, what is more important to spend your money on, that daily specialty coffee, a bigger TV, more channels on your cable or satellite TV, having your nails done or protecting you and your family from chemicals, additives, antibiotics, and growth hormones in your food that may eventually have horrible repercussions like cancer? The good news is since awareness of the dangers of these products in our foods has been heightened and more people are choosing organic, major grocery store chains are jumping on the bandwagon and selling more and more organic foods and at much better price points than specialty health stores. My advice? Do your best to buy the fruits and vegetables on the dirty dozen list organic, buy all other fruits and vegetable USA grown and when organic or antibiotic/steroid free pork, poultry and beef products go on sale (which happens a lot in the major chain grocery stores) stock up!! Freeze it!! Dairy should be organic or hormone free as often as possible too.   Pork and poultry products are already hormone free as there are no approved growth hormones for these products. Labeling claiming pork or poultry products as "hormone free" may be trying to get you to pay more for something you would be getting anyway with all pork and chicken products. However "organic" labeling on pork and poultry products would insure they were free of antibiotics too.

So, YES! Buy organic...............wisely!

BODYINSTINCT "6 WEEK TOTAL TRANSFORMATION PROGRAM"

WEEK 2
FITNESS GUIDELINES:

<u>**Strength/resistance training program**</u>: Do some type of strength training such as Hard-Body Yoga™, Pilates or weightlifting for 30-60 minutes twice a week.

<u>**Cardio program**</u>: Three 20-minute cardio workouts a week done very intensely in an interval fashion. 4 minutes at or above your 75% range and the 5th minute at full blast then repeat this 4 times total to complete 20 minutes. Warm up and cool down do not count towards the 20 minutes. A heart rate monitor is highly recommended to make sure you are burning fat most efficiently. (to find your 75% range: 220 – your age x 75%) **Do your cardio first thing in the morning on an empty stomach or immediately after your weight/resistance workout.**

NUTRITION PROGRAM EATING INSTINCTS:

- <u>**Eating Instinct #1:**</u> Eat unprocessed foods whenever possible (food in its natural state). Your diet should consist mainly of lean high quality protein, fruits & vegetables.
- <u>**Eating Instinct #2:**</u> Eat with your Circadian rhythm. Be a daytime eater. Always eat breakfast, make lunch your main meal, and think of dinner as a small light meal, consisting of lean protein and vegetables.

- **Eating Instinct #3:** NEVER let more than 3 hours go by without food. Eat several small meals instead of 2-3 big ones or supplement 3 regular meals with healthy unprocessed snacks such as fruit, veggies or nuts in between.
- **Eating Instinct #4:** Avoid most saturated fat and **all** hydrogenated oils (trans fats). The fat in your diet should be coming mostly from nuts, seeds, olives, and avocados. (oils should be used sparingly and should be cold or expeller pressed) Remove all products with hydrogenated or partially hydrogenated oils from your home.
- **Eating Instinct #5:** Drink at least **64** oz. (8 cups) of water every day.
- **Eating Instinct #6:** Make sure you are getting lean high quality protein at least 3 times a day.
- **Eating Instinct #7:** Avoid eating after 7:00 pm or 12 hours after regular wake up time.
- **Eating Instinct #8: Restrict energy foods: nuts & seeds, fruit and especially starchy carbs (rice, pasta, bread, sugar, potatoes, and flour products) after 3:00 pm. You are what you eat after 3:00 pm!**
- **Eating Instinct #9: Limit alcohol intake to no more than 1 glass of wine or beer a day. (7 glasses a week).**
- **Eating Instinct #10: Don't drink your calories! This includes fruit & vegetable juices. Eat the whole fruit or vegetable instead!**

CHAPTER TWO:

THE BALL IS ROLLING!

WEEK TWO

FITNESS GUIDELINES:

Creating a lean strong body with strength training!

<u>Strength/resistance training program</u>: *Creating a lean strong fat burning body!!* **Do some type of strength/resistance training such as Hard-Body Yoga™, Pilates or weightlifting for 30-60 minutes twice a week.**

Now that you have a week of BodyInstinct style cardio under your belt it's time to add strength training. If you were already doing strength training and so graciously resisted the temptation to engage in it last week as requested, you're probably chomping at the bit to get back into it! If you've never done any type of strength training before or not for a very long time, don't worry! There's something for everyone! Just as in our discussion on the various types of cardio exercise, strength training has no one superior method! There are sculpting classes, Pilates, weight machines, free weights, toning classes, even my own personal concoction Hard-Body Yoga™ (a blend of Pilates and yoga)! You can join a gym, a class or rent a video. You can even do your resistance training in the comforts of your own home with no special equipment, videos or even electricity! The important thing is to pick something that you like doing and do it!

Strength training is defined as: *the use of resistance to muscular contraction to build the strength, anaerobic endurance and size/tone of skeletal muscles.* The resistance can come from dumbbells, machines, elastic bands or even your own body weight (my favorite and the safest and most effective method!) Why is it important to do strength training? Stronger muscles, stronger bones, better posture, and increased fat burning! Many people avoid resistance training in favor of more cardio workouts thinking they would rather spend their workout time burning calories. Well, that's exactly what they get. They burn calories *during* their workout time. But what about the other 23+ hours of the day??? Wouldn't you like to be burning more calories then??? You will if you are strength/resistance training! Strength/resistance training increases your muscle density, size and tone which increases your resting metabolic rate. In other words, by increasing the size, density and tone of your muscles, you burn more calories throughout the whole day. Even when you are just sitting at the computer or watching TV. Your cardio workout does a great job burning fat and calories *while* you are doing it but your strength training workout helps you to burn more calories and fat all day every day!

You may know someone who goes to the gym 5 or 6 days a week and weight trains different body parts on different days or maybe someone who does 3 or 4 sculpting or Pilate's classes a week. Once again, these people are overtraining and less would be more. The act itself of doing a sculpting class or a weight training session does not make your muscles bigger, stronger or more toned. The strength/resistance workout itself is actually breaking down the muscle. The rest period in between workouts is when your body is reaping the benefits of your resistance training. Your muscles are recovering and building back stronger, with more density, tone and size preparing themselves for your next workout.

This brings us to your new recommendations for your strength/resistance training workout: workout your whole body twice a week for 30 to 60 minutes. This style of training your muscles gives you exactly what you need to be fit, strong and healthy with plenty of recovery time in between workouts! Also, if you do the math: strength training twice a week for 30 to 60 minutes + 3-20 minute cardio sessions = 2 to 3 hours a week *total* spent on your fitness program. Now that's doable and something that you can continue for the rest of your life with no problem. Maximum results, minimum time invested!

For those of you who have no idea what type of strength/resistance training workout to do, or if you need something that is simple and effective yet you can do at home or anywhere with no special equipment at all, I have included the basic resistance training workout for you! Actually, this workout is great for everybody! You can call it your "no excuses" workout because it is available for you to do anytime anywhere: in a hotel room, park, at the beach, or in your living room in your underwear! The other great part is you need no special equipment, no weights, no bands, no balls, not even electricity! Even shoes are optional! Let's take a look:

BodyInstinct Basic resistance training workout:

Squats (with or without weights)
    2 sets of 20 reps
with feet planted on ground a little wider than shoulder width apart and arms straight out in front at shoulder level (unless you are holding weights then your arms would be at your sides), bend knees and squat down as low as you personally can go with the lowest being when the tops of your thighs are parallel to the floor. Press back up pushing through heels and squeezing your butt. Repeat 20 times, rest briefly and do one more set of 20. It is important to remember when doing these squats or any squats to keep the majority of your weight in your heels to avoid overtaxing the knees and to get more exercise for your butt, lower back and backs of legs. If you are a beginner or have not worked out recently, start with one

set of 10 repetitions and work your way up, adding additional reps/sets each time until you are doing 2 sets of 20. Move up at your own pace.

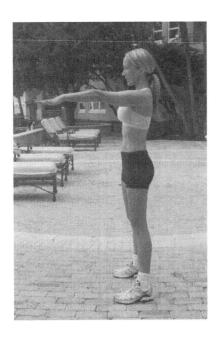 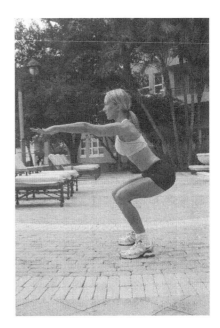

Dips off of chair
   3 sets of 10 reps

*any chair or sturdy surface such as a side of a bathtub will do. As long as the height falls between 1-3 feet. The higher the easier, the lower the more challenging. Sit on the chair or sturdy object with your hands on the chair or object right next to your hips with your fingers curled over the front side. Steadying yourself with your arms Remove your butt from the chair, shift slightly forward to clear the chair and walk your feet out a little. With your knees bent and your feet either flat on the floor with your ankles directly under your knees (easier version) or straightened legs out in front of you resting on heels with toes pointed up, slowly lower yourself until your shoulders are even with your elbows. Push back up to start. Repeat for 10 repetitions then rest briefly and perform two more sets. If you are a beginner or have never done this exercise before I would recommend you start with one set of 6 – 10 repetitions and work your way up.

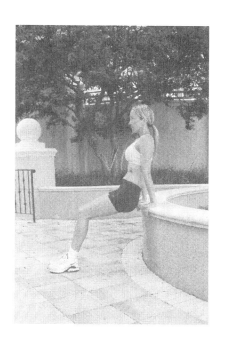 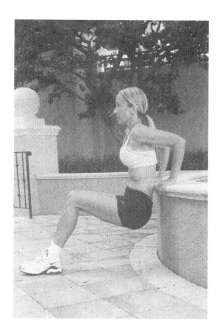

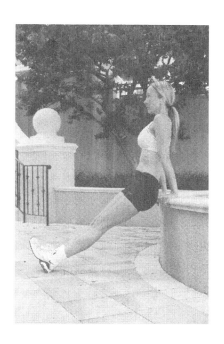 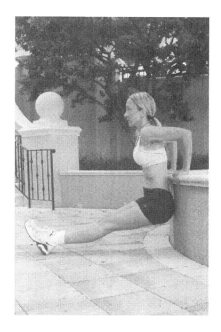

Backward lunges

2 sets of 20 each leg (do all 20 on same side then switch sides)
Place feet together standing alone or holding on with one hand to a chair or sturdy surface for balance. Reach back with your right leg as if you were going to kneel on the floor into a lunge. In the beginning you can just do a small bend but eventually your back knee should feather touch the floor. Press through the heel of the front foot to bring you back up to start. Repeat up to 20 times on the same side with the same leg. Rest until your breath becomes normal and repeat on the other leg. Rest again and repeat once more on each leg. If you are a beginner or haven't worked out in a while I would start with just one set of 10 on each leg and work your way up.

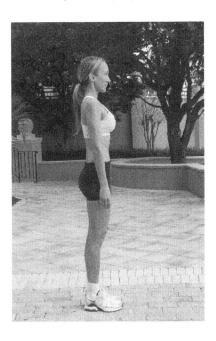 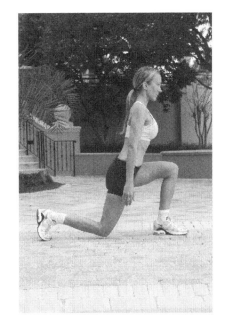

Pushups

3 sets of 10 reps (do regular, on knees, or on a sturdy table, wall or bench)
Start either in regular push up position or on your hands and knees with a straight body. Being slow and controlled and leading with your chest,

lower yourself a little or a lot depending on your fitness level. The farthest down you should go is one fist length from the floor. Push back up to start. If you are a beginner, I would start with one set of 6-10 repetitions and work up to 3 sets. Before attempting regular pushups make sure you can do three sets of 10 of the bent knee pushups with great form and full range of motion.

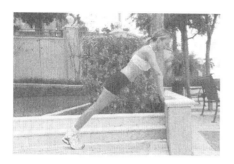
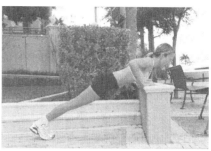

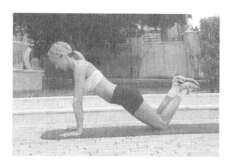
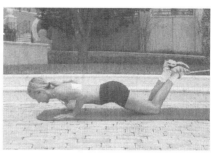

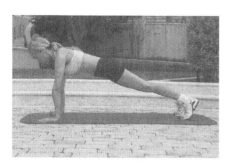
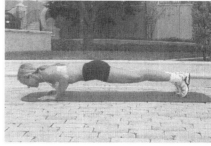

Bridging

2 sets of 20 reps

Start lying on your back on the floor with arms at your sides and knees bent with feet comfortably close to your butt and comfortably apart from each other (about hip width or wider). Pushing through your heels, lift torso off floor and push up as high as you can go lifting as much of your spine off the floor as possible. Slowly lower back down and feather touch the floor with your butt then push back up. Beginners should probably start with 2 sets of 10 repetitions and work their way up to 2 sets of 20 repetitions.

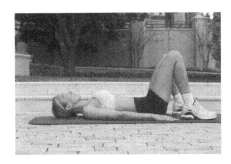 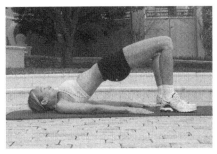

Abs

3 sets of 50 of the following

-elbows to knees

-reverse crunches

-twisting elbows to knees

The most important part of doing abdominal exercises (abs) is doing them correctly. 10 repetitions done correctly are worth more than 100 repetitions done poorly. You want to think quality instead of quantity. The way to get quality ab work is to engage your transverse abdominus or the paper thin muscle that runs behind your rectus abdominus (the 6 pack). You don't see the transverse abdominus but it's the muscle that does the majority of the job of holding your stomach in and flat. The best way to work the transverse abdominus is isometrically or by "pulling it in". If you do abdominal exercises without pulling in your stomach the whole time, you will not affect your transverse and will not achieve a flatter stomach.

You will just hit your rectus abdominus which is mainly responsible for trunk flexion but doesn't do too much to pull your stomach in flatter. That being said, during your abdominal repetitions, you want to be pulling your belly button in towards your spine and pressing your spine down into the floor taking the curve out of your lower back as much as possible. When you can maintain the lower back pressing down and into the floor while doing your ab exercises, you will truly be working your transverse abdominus and be on your way to a flatter stomach. You will also notice that your ab work becomes harder and more challenging with your transverse abdominus engaged. That's because you are doing them correctly.

The 3 exercises I have included in this workout are basic abdominal exercises. Let's go over them:

1. *Elbows to knees – start in a lying down position on your back. Knees are bent with feet on the floor close to your butt. Finger tips are behind your head for support (resist the temptation to clasp hands behind your head). Pulling in the stomach and keeping the lower back down pressed into the floor, raise head and feet off the floor at the same time bringing elbows and knees together or as close as possible. (If this is too difficult at first you can lift only one knee in each time alternating.) Keep a tennis ball space between your chin and your chest to avoid pulling on your neck. As you lower back down to start remember to keep the stomach pulled in and the lower back pressed into the floor. Maintain this pulled in position the entire time. Start with 10-15 repetitions and work your way up to 50.*

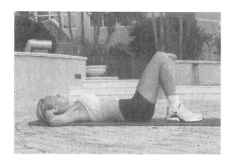 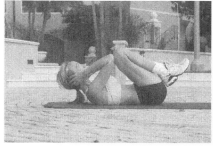

2. *Reverse crunches – start in a lying down position on your back with your knees bent and feet close to your butt on the floor. Pull in stomach pressing lower back down and into the floor. While maintaining this pulled in position, lift knees into chest while curling tailbone up off of the floor and then bring heels back down to floor keeping stomache tight, pulled in and lower back pressed down into floor. Start with 10-15 repetitions and work your way up to 50.*

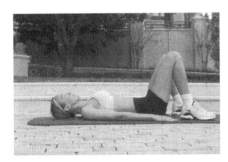 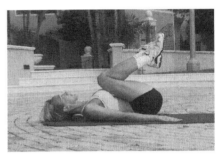

3. *Twisting elbows to knees (this exercise incorporates your waist muscles or obliques. The thing about working obliques is you always want to work them by moving across your body during abs in a lying down position, NEVER do standing twisting exercises, or side bends. These types of waist exercises are guaranteed to make your waist bigger by increasing the size of your obliques and pushing the fat on your waist out even further. Working your waist in the way that I am about to suggest has more of a "cinching" effect on your waist, pulling it in smaller and tighter.)– start in the same position as ab exercise #1. This time when you lift up to bring elbows and knees together, do a little twist to one side bringing the right elbow to the outside of the left knee, come back down and on your next repetition do a little twist to the other side bringing the left elbow to the outside of the right knee. If this is too difficult at first, you can lift just one leg off the floor twisting upper body and bringing the opposite elbow to the outside of that knee and then lower and repeat on the other side. Start with 10-15 repetitions and work up to 50.*

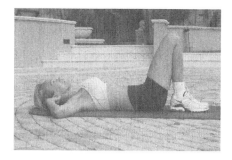 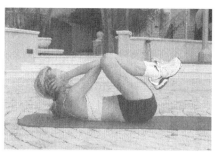

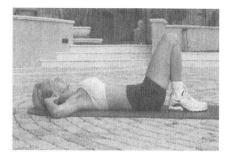 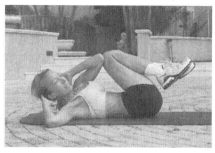

Cardio Program: *The best time to exercise to burn the most fat!* **Do your cardio first thing in the morning on an empty stomach or immediately after your weight/resistance workout.**

In week one you implemented your 3 cardio workouts done in an interval fashion. Now, in week two without changing anything about your cardio except *when* you do it, we can increase your fat burning efficiency by 200%! That's right! Timing is everything when it comes to cardio! As far as the amount of fat you will burn, 20 minutes first thing in the morning on an empty stomach is equivalent to doing 60 minutes any other time of day! That should be enough convincing to get you up and out of bed just 20 minutes earlier only 3 days a week! Let's talk a little bit about why you burn so much more fat doing your cardio first thing in the morning on an empty stomach:

All food that is consumed is turned into glucose in the bloodstream and then burned or converted into one of two stored fuel sources in your body: glycogen or fat. Glycogen is the bodies most easily accessible and most preferred stored fuel source. Glycogen is stored mainly in your muscles and fat is stored mainly....well.....pretty much everywhere else. Normally, when you do a cardio workout, your body burns a combination of glycogen and fat as fuel. The advantage to doing your cardio first thing in the morning on an empty stomach is that when you wake up in the morning your glycogen energy system is depleted. The glycogen storage in your muscles is *very* low and you also haven't eaten in hours (hopefully 12) so there is no food roaming around in your bloodstream (glucose) to be burned while you exercise either. The only thing you have plenty of to burn is fat! This is why the percentage of fat burned during cardio exercise is the highest first thing in the morning on an empty stomach.

It's perfectly ok if you want to hydrate with plain old water. No flavored waters or bubbled waters or water with lemon. Just water. If the idea of water jostling around in your stomach doesn't sound comfortable you definitely don't have to drink it. If you met your mandatory water consumption the day before, you will be hydrated.

If it is totally physically impossible for you to get up and do cardio first thing in the morning on an empty stomach, the second best time is immediately following your strength/resistance training. Your body uses glycogen almost exclusively for strength/resistance training so when you are finished training your muscles you have very little glycogen left. Once again you will be burning a very high percentage of fat since that is pretty much all you have left to burn. Although this is the second best time to burn fat doing cardio, it still doesn't come close to doing your cardio right out of bed on an empty stomach.

Another advantage to doing cardio first thing in the morning is it's over and done with and a great way to start your day with a healthy body and a healthy attitude!

WEEK TWO ADDITIONAL EATING INSTINCTS:

*Note: water intake increases to 64 oz. (8 cups)

*<u>Eating Instinct #8:</u> *You are what you eat – after 3:00 pm!!*

Restrict energy foods: nuts & seeds, fruit and especially starchy carbs (rice, pasta, bread, sugar, potatoes, and flour products) after 3:00 pm.

The old saying "you are what you eat" is only partially true. "You are what you eat after 3:00 pm" is my revised edition of the old saying and is the real truth!

If you could take only one thing from this program and implement it to change your life drastically, this is it! I have been practicing this for over 20 years with myself and my clients and it is fail proof! Eating more, earlier in the day and strictly limiting calories after 3 is a quick easy, painless way to a leaner body! It's magical!

The best example I have of how great this concept works is the following story: I was once taking a client on a "healthy shopping trip" in the grocery store, pointing out and explaining healthy food choices. I was also enlightening them about the 3:00 pm eating instinct and was not aware that an employee of the grocery store was listening. Two months later I was in that same grocery store again and that employee came up to me hugged me, and thanked me for my overheard advice. Just by implementing the after 3:00 pm rule, he had lost 16 pounds! And that was the only advice he had heard!

Start by considering foods to be in two food groups: energy foods and repair and recovery foods:

<u>Energy Foods</u> - nuts & seeds, fruit and starchy carbs (rice, pasta, bread, sugar, potatoes, and all flour products whether whole grain or not)

Repair & Recovery Foods – vegetables and proteins

Energy foods are exactly what the name implies compact get up and go higher calorie foods with amazing nutrients that you need to be eating when your body is expending the most energy: during the day and before 3:00 pm! Repair and recovery foods are foods that are super high in the nutrients, antioxidants and vitamins and minerals that your body needs to start repairing the damage done at the cellular level in your body each day.

It really is the foods you eat later in the day that determine what your body looks (and feels) like. I guarantee you it's the food you have been eating after 3:00 pm that is sticking to your waist line. If you stick to eating only vegetables and lean proteins after 3:00 pm, you will be amazed at how fast your body changes! To reiterate, this means no energy foods: nuts & seeds, fruit, and especially starchy carbs (rice, pasta, bread, sugar, potatoes, and flour products) after 3:00 pm. It's important to know that the BodyInstinct program is *not* anti-carb. Low/no carb diets have been around for decades and they certainly don't work or everyone would be skinny by now. Carbs (aka energy foods) are very important to your body and your brain. If you have ever tried one of the low/no carb diets I'm sure you've had the experience of lightheadedness, low energy, inability to concentrate and irritability. Carbs are not the enemy. They are full of fiber and nutrients that your body needs. However, carbs *are* calorically dense energy foods as are nuts, fruits and seeds and should be eaten during the early part of the day when you are expending the most energy. If you do not eat adequate amounts of energy foods during the day, you will be starving by evening and over-eat….period. Eat those energy foods during the day and abstain after 3 pm!

If you've ever noticed, right around 2 or 3 pm in the middle of the day, you get a little tired slump. What that is actually, is your circadian rhythm causing a big drop in your body's metabolism for the rest of the day. Most people just grab a cup of coffee or tea at this point and push past it. What they really should be doing is paying attention to what their body is trying to say. "I am slowing down and will be burning very few calories for the rest of the day. I am going into repair and recovery mode and I need modest amounts of repair and recovery food NOT energy food! If you give me energy food, I will only store it as fat somewhere on your body that you will not appreciate".

Hopefully, you have already been implementing last weeks eating instinct #2 – Eat with your circadian rhythm and be a day-time eater! That was introduced into week one to get your feet wet with the idea and slowly introduce your body to the concept. Now in week two it's time for you to make the complete transition into a daytime eater. To make that transition seamless and easy you have to continue to eat for energy before 3 pm so that you are not starving after 3 pm making it very difficult to eat a small dinner of lean protein and vegetables. Eat a substantial breakfast and lunch with a snack in between and another snack right around that 3:00 pm time. Then when dinner time comes it is easy to eat a modest amount of protein and vegetables.

Choosing protein and vegetables for dinner every night does not have to be boring. In fact, it can be downright fun and delicious! You can have anything from the protein list at the end of chapter one and anything from the vegetable list. Ok, still not excited? Well think like this:

Monday: grilled chicken breast marinated in Balsamic dressing with grilled asparagus with a little olive oil and coarse salt and a side of Greek salad.

Tuesday: blackened salmon with steamed or frozen brussel sprouts and corn.

Wednesday: out to your favorite local bar and grill for hot chicken wings naked (the wings not you) and lots of celery and carrot sticks (easy on the blue cheese)

Thursday: throw a steak on the grill with an ear of corn and some sliced zucchini or a tomato and onion salad with Italian dressing

Friday: out to your favorite Mexican restaurant for chicken, steak or shrimp fajitas minus the tortillas! Just put the guaca-mole and salsa and a little cheese if you choose right on top of the sizzling fajitas and eat up!

Saturday: Lean pork chops, sour kraut, and cooked carrots and peas

Sunday: at a birthday party where the only food is pizza. No worries! You can just eat the cheese and toppings and leave the dough behind or go ahead and have a whole slice. You have made great choices all week long and just this one night of en-ergy foods after 3 is not going to reverse all the good! Although, you may regret it later for other reasons. (More to come on that)

The key is to think delicious and fun instead of deprived! As you can see by the dinners above, it is a good idea to sometimes have more than one vegetable choice so that your chicken breast and broccoli don't look so lonely and boring sitting there on your plate! Add that side salad or sliced tomatoes! If you are wondering about salad dressings it's easy: any dressing is acceptable used in modest amounts. If you are making the salad, then add a very small amount to the whole salad (like a tablespoon for a big bowl or a teaspoon for a small bowl for one) and toss toss toss! Make that little bit of dressing go a long way! If you are eating out in a restaurant, DON'T tell them to put the dressing on the side. You will definitely use more than if you had let them put it on because you have no means to toss that salad and really spread it through. Instead, ask them to please go very light on the dressing. They will toss it through and that way you get less dressing but the taste of it on every bite!

Although fruits, nuts and seeds are energy foods, it's ok to have them as "accents" in your dinner. Example: some mandarin oranges, walnuts, or sunflower seeds in your salad. Or peanuts in your stir fry. As long as these energy foods are in small amounts and used more as an accent you are doing ok. What you strictly want to stay away from is the starchy carbs such as sugar, rice, bread, potatoes and pasta. Whole grain or refined, it doesn't matter. They are still energy foods and should be reserved for before 3 pm. Even a little bit of these foods can set off a carbohydrate binge. Most people do not have the willpower to eat just a bite of these foods mainly because it's just not about willpower. There is an actual physiological response that happens when you ingest starchy carbs that encourages you to eat more starchy carbs so best to stay away from them completely after 3 pm.

After practicing the after 3pm instinct for a week or so, your body's natural instincts will kick back in and you will automatically begin to reject energy foods late in the day. On the occasion that you do indulge in energy foods late in the day (as I suggested in the eating example for Sunday) you will suddenly be very aware of them in your system. You will find it very difficult to sleep, tossing, turning and sweating and you will most likely wake up with what feels like a mild hangover. All just more proof energy foods are not meant to be eaten late in the day. The loss of a good nights sleep is also a very effective way of deterring you from consuming energy foods late in the day very often!

*Eating Instinct #9: *Alcohol and your health.* **Limit alcohol intake to no more than 1 glass of wine or beer a day. (7 glasses a week)**

You may have seen studies or heard that people who drink red wine are healthier than people who don't. The argument is for a few reasons. First of all moderate consumption of alcohol in general (not just red wine) has been shown to raise your healthy "good" cholesterol (HDL), lower blood pressure and prevent blood clots. In addition, research at Texas Tech University Health Services has shown that individuals drinking one drink a day are 54% less likely to have a weight problem.

Wine, specifically red wine, is a rich source of polyphenol antioxidants including phenolics, flavonoids, and resveratrol. These antioxidants prevent cellular damage caused by free radicals which can lead to heart disease and cancer. They are found primarily in the skins and peels of fruit. White wines have their

skins removed before being placed into vats for fermentation giving them a lower concentration of polyphenols than red. New
research on resveratrol has shown it may slow down the aging
process.

The American Heart Association recommends limiting alcohol to one drink a day for women and 1-2 drinks a day for men.
A "drink" is considered to be one 12 oz beer, 4 oz. of wine, or
1 oz of spirits.

On the other hand, consuming 3 or more drinks a day de-
creases the body's ability to burn fat and suppresses the hormone
leptin which tells you when you are full. Drinking more alcohol
also increases such dangers as alcoholism, high blood pressure,
obesity, stroke, breast cancer, suicide and accidents. Once again
it's a true tale of "everything in moderation" and yet another dis-
claimer for the huge health misconception: "if a little is good for
you then a lot must be better".

Also, it's not possible to predict in which people alcoholism
will become a problem. For these and other risk factors I cau-
tion people NOT to start drinking ... if you do not already drink
alcohol.

However, if you already do consume alcohol, for the purposes
of the BodyInstinct program, we are going to make sure you are
drinking no more than 7 drinks a week. I have found in my experience with good health and nutrition that is what you do to
and with your body over the course of a week that is important.
As long as during one whole week you have created balance in
your body, you are on track. For this reason, if you prefer to have
a couple of drinks on the weekend nights instead of spreading
your alcohol consumption evenly throughout the week, that's
fine just as long as you are drinking responsibly and you don't go
over 7 drinks in the course of the entire week.

I also prefer that you consume either wine or beer, limiting
consumption of hard alcohol or spirits for special occasions. It's
not so much the liquor that is the problem but most people mix

it with juice, soda or other mixers and that adds a lot of calories and sugar. This brings us to our next eating instinct:

*Eating Instinct #10: *Don't drink your calories!* **This includes fruit & vegetable juices. Eat the whole fruit or vegetable instead!**

There is a huge problem in this country with drinking our calories. With super size containers for sodas, coffee, and smoothies, you can easily drink more than 1000 calories a day! That of course is in addition to the food you are already eating. Let's look at the calorie count of some popular beverages:

Soda
- Soda (20-oz bottle) = 250 calories (that is 5.8 tablespoons of sugar!)
- 7/11 Big Gulp (32-oz) = 400 calories (8.9 tablespoons of sugar!)
- 7/11 Double Big Gulp (64-oz) = 800 calories (17.7 tablespoons of sugar!)
  100% of the calories in soda are from sugar!!!

Tea and Coffee Drinks
- Arizona Lemon Iced Tea (16-oz bottle) = 180 calories (4 tablespoons of sugar) 100% of the calories are from sugar!!!
- Starbucks Mocha Frappuccino® (with whip):
  - Tall (12-oz) = 270 calories (3½ tablespoons of sugar)
  - Grande (16-oz) = 370 calories (4 tablespoons + 2 tsp sugar)
  - Venti (24-oz) = 470 calories (6½ tablespoons of sugar)

More than 58% of the calories in these drinks come from sugar!!! Flavored hot coffees such as the White Chocolate Mocha are just about the same or worse as Frappuccinos® as far as calories and sugar and don't think you are doing yourself any favors by ordering the Starbucks Chai Tea Latte. That too is high in sugar.

Fruit Beverages and smoothies

Jamba Juice Banana Berry (classic smoothie):
- 16-oz = 270 calories (5 tablespoons of sugar)
- 24-oz original = 400 calories (7.3 tablespoons of sugar)
- 30-oz power = 560 calories (10.2 tablespoons of sugar)

Over 80% of the calories in this smoothie comes from sugar!

- POM Pomegranate Juice (16-oz bottle) = 320 calories (over 6 tablespoons of sugar) 85% of calories from sugar
- Orange Juice (pint container, 16-oz) = 220 calories (3.7 tablespoons of sugar) 76% of calories from sugar

Flavored Waters and Sports Drinks

- Vitamin Water (20-oz bottle) = 125 calories (2.9 tablespoons of sugar) 100% of calories from sugar
- Gatorade (20-oz bottle) = 125 calories (3.1 tablespoons of sugar)
  100% of calories from sugar

In all of these beverages the majority if not all of their calories are coming from sugar! Some people would argue that fruit juice is good for you and therefore should not be grouped in with these sugary drinks. The truth is "fruit" is good for you and if you ate the whole fruit instead of drinking just the juice you would be better off as far as lower sugar intake, higher fiber intake and more antioxidants. Let's look at orange juice to make our point: one 16 oz container of orange juice has 42 grams of sugar and 220 calories. How many oranges do you think it takes to make this one container of juice? Anywhere between 4 and 5 depending on the size of the oranges. Now, would you ever sit down and eat 4 or 5 oranges in one sitting? Probably not, but if you did , you would be consuming all of the fiber that was intended by nature to be eaten with the sugary juice which would slow down the absorption of that sugar into your bloodstream and make it more likely the sugar would be burned up as energy instead of stored as fat. Without that fiber all the sugar from the orange juice is rushing into your system all at once. Think about it. If you know someone who is a diabetic you know that when a diabetic has too much insulin in their system and their blood sugar gets too low, they need to get sugar into their bloodstream as quickly as possible. How are they told to do it? Eat a cookie? Eat a candy bar? NO. They are told to get the most sugar into their bloodstream the fastest they should drink juice.

Juice fanatics may argue too that you get more antioxidants vitamins and minerals by juicing many fruits or vegetables instead of just eating a few. The truth is most fruits and vegetables contain valuable nutrients in the skins, peels and membranes. Let's once again take orange juice as an example: one single orange has 5 times more of one major anti-oxidant than a glass of orange juice. This antioxidant is found in the membranes that separate the orange segments from each other. That part is left behind in the juicing process.

What to do if you just LOVE smoothies and shakes and you just can't live without them? Make your own or have your favorite juice place make them your way. Put the *whole* fruit or vegetable into the blender and add just enough water to make it liquid. There is a great recipe for the BodyInstinct Shake at the back of this book in the recipe section! Give it a try!

THE BODYINSTINCT ONE SHEET EATING PLAN

I used the BodyInstinct Program for many years with my clients before I ever implemented the BodyInstinct One Sheet Eating Plan. I was asked by many people to please structure the program so they would know exactly what to eat and exactly when to eat it. I resisted for some time believing that too much structure is not always a good thing and can send someone running in the opposite direction. On the other hand, some of my type "A" clients and friends (and you know who you are) said they thrive on structure and would be more successful with a little more. This is for those of you that want to be told exactly what to eat and exactly when to eat it. Use this one sheet structured eating plan in conjunction with the BodyInstinct Food Source pages found at the end of Chapter One (Protein, Starchy Carbs, Vegetables, Fruit, Fats). Any time you are following the BodyInstinct One Sheet Eating Plan exactly, you are doing the eating part of the program 100%. If you do not want to follow the structured eating plan and would rather get into more of a groove of your own yet stay within the Eating Instinct guidelines, that's fine. However, I do recommend that sometime during week 2 everyone follows the One Sheet Eating Plan for at least 1 day so you have a very clear idea of what a 100% day is like.

BODYINSTINCT STRUCTURED EATING PLAN

Meal one breakfast
Choose 1 protein source
Choose 1 starchy carb source

Snack
Choose 1 fruit source (e.g. any 1 whole fruit or 1 cup)
Choose ½ fat source (e.g. ½ your handful of nuts)

Meal two lunch
Choose 1 protein source
Choose 1 starchy carb source

Snack (must be eaten by 3:00 pm)
Choose 1 fruit source (e.g. any 1 whole fruit or 1 cup)
Choose ½ fat source (e.g. ½ your handful of nuts)

Meal three dinner
Choose 1 protein source + veggies

NOTE: A starchy carb source can be replaced by the following:
½ starchy carb source + 1 fruit source
OR
2 fruit sources

*veggies are unlimited all day long

Remember to refer to your "Food Source" sheets for
appropriate food choices and serving size.

BODYINSTINCT "6 WEEK TOTAL TRANSFORMATION PROGRAM"

WEEK 3
FITNESS GUIDELINES:

<u>**Weight/resistance training program**</u>: Do some type of resistance training such as Hard-Body Yoga™, pilates or weightlifting for 30-60 minutes twice a week.

<u>**Cardio program**</u>: Three 20-minute cardio workouts a week done very intensely in an interval fashion. 4 minutes at or above your 75% range and the 5th minute at full blast then repeat this 4 times total to complete 20 minutes. Warm up and cool down do not count towards the 20 minutes. A heart rate monitor is highly recommended to make sure you are burning fat most efficiently. (to find your 75% range: 220 – your age x 75%) Do your cardio first thing in the morning on an empty stomach or immediately after your weight/resistance workout. **Whenever possible, wait one hour after cardio before eating.**

NUTRITION PROGRAM EATING INSTINCTS:

- <u>**Eating Instinct #1:**</u> Eat unprocessed foods whenever possible (food in its natural state). Your diet should consist mainly of lean high quality protein, fruits & vegetables.
- <u>**Eating Instinct #2:**</u> Be a daytime eater. Always eat breakfast, make lunch your main meal, and think of dinner as a small light meal consisting of lean protein and vegetables.

- **Eating Instinct #3:** NEVER let more than 3 hours go by without food. Eat several small meals instead of 2-3 big ones or supplement 3 regular meals with healthy unprocessed snacks such as fruit, veggies or nuts in between.
- **Eating Instinct #4:** Avoid most saturated fat and **all** hydrogenated oils (trans fats). The fat in your diet should be coming mostly from nuts, seeds, olives, and avocados. (oils should be used sparingly and should be cold or expeller pressed) Remove all products with hydrogenated or partially hydrogenated oils from your home.
- **Eating Instinct #5:** Drink at least **80** oz. (10 cups) of water every day.
- **Eating Instinct #6:** Make sure you are getting lean high quality protein at least 3 times a day.
- **Eating Instinct #7:** Avoid eating after 7:00 pm or 12 hours after regular wake up time.
- **Eating Instinct #8:** Restrict energy foods: nuts & seeds, fruit and especially starchy carbs (rice, pasta, bread, sugar, potatoes, and flour products) after 3:00 pm. You are what you eat after 3:00 pm!
- **Eating Instinct #9:** Limit alcohol intake to no more than 1 glass of wine or beer a day. (7 glasses a week)
- **Eating Instinct #10:** Don't drink your calories! This includes fruit & vegetable juices. Eat the whole fruit or vegetable instead!
- **Eating Instinct #11: Restrict refined sugars and sweet snacks. (if desired you may have ONE small sweet snack per day before 3:00 pm) Do not keep ANY sweets in your house.**
- **Eating Instinct #12: Do your best to get 7-8 hours sleep a night.**
- **Eating Instinct #13: Take one brand name multiple vitamin daily such as Centrum or One a Day.**

CHAPTER THREE

YOUR INSTINCTS KICKING BACK IN!

WEEK THREE

FITNESS GUIDELINES:

How would you like an extra 3 hours of fatburning with no exertion on your part?

Strength and Resistance program: Remains the same

Cardio Program: *Time can be on your side!* **Whenever possible wait one hour after cardio before eating.**

I have yet one more little trick up my sleeve when it comes to getting the most out of your cardio. Waiting an hour after your cardio workout before you eat is a great way to burn even more fat without exerting yourself at all! When you finish your cardio, your metabolism continues to race for about an hour afterwards burning additional calories. If you keep your stomach empty during that time (plain water of course is always ok) you will have nothing available to burn but body fat. If you drink or eat something with calories, your body will start to convert those ingested calories into fuel to be burned instead of burning your body fat. Especially if you drink a sugary drink or shake. When you are through with your cardio, drink a glass of plain water to re-hydrate and help you to burn that extra body fat then take your shower or check your email or do something to delay your eating for an hour. As always, "a little is good a lot must be better" does not apply here either. Waiting beyond an hour to eat will actually begin to slow your metabolism down. You need to eat somewhere within that hour. If you can only wait a half an hour, so be it. Just remember that the closer you get to that full hour the more body fat you will burn. Keep in mind that if you practice this concept after all three of your weekly cardio workouts, you will get an additional 3 hours of body fat burning each week!

WEEK THREE ADDITIONAL EATING INSTINCTS:

*Note: water intake increases to 80 oz. (10 cups) a day

*Eating Instinct #11: *Satisfy your sweet tooth without sabotaging your body!* Restrict refined sugars and sweet snacks. (If desired you may have ONE small sweet snack per day before 3:00 pm) Do not keep ANY sweets in your house.

There are three types of people when it comes to sugar:
Type A: This person needs just a little sweet treat every day. One small cookie or a piece of chocolate is all they need to satisfy their craving and they are fine. If they don't have it they feel as if they are missing something and start to do what I call "eating around the craving". Which means, to avoid eating the sweet, they eat everything else they can think of that is healthy in hopes of the craving going away. Then when it doesn't go away, they end up eating the sweet too. Now, if they would have just eaten a small sweet when they originally had the craving, they could have saved

themselves a lot of extra calories trying to avoid it. Lesson learned: never eat around a craving. Also remember if you are this type, have your daily sweet treat before 3:00 pm because sugar is an energy food and energy foods need to be eaten before 3! In fact you should replace one of your two snacks with the healthiest sweet treat you can get your hands on such as the BodyInstinct Banana Bread/Muffins in the recipe section at the back of this book. Or ½ of a peanut butter and jelly sandwich on whole wheat. Or 1 VitaTops 100 calorie Muffin tops which come in many varieties including chocolate which are really yummy!! Or if it's just a smaller treat you need, have a small piece (1 inch square) of dark chocolate or 5 dark chocolate M&M's or 1 hershey's kiss after lunch.

Type B: This person cannot even think about eating just one cookie or one piece of chocolate. It's the whole bag or box or nothing!! Obviously, for this person it needs to be nothing. One reason this person might exhibit this "all or nothing" behavior when it comes to sweets is this: They may actually be physically addicted to sugar. In our intestines live yeast (or candida). The favorite food of these yeast organisms is sugar. The more sugar you eat, the more the yeast multiplies and then you have more yeast wanting more sugar. Your body physically needs the sugar to feed the yeast otherwise they die off which they certainly don't want to do. To break this cycle of more and more yeast needing more and more sugar, you need to stay away from sugar as much as possible. That is why this type B person needs to abstain from sugary treats completely at least for a couple of weeks until some of that yeast dies off. At that time a type B can try just eating one cookie and see how it goes. If it sets off a binge, then they need to abstain from sugar for a couple more weeks and try again. Another problem with a lot of yeast is it creates bloating that can counteract your efforts of trying to get a flat stomach. Bloating yeast is stronger than any abdominal exercise out there!

Type C: This person could care less about sweets whatsoever. If a type C is overweight it is usually because fatty foods and white flour processed salty foods are their vice.

Regardless of what type you are, sweets should NEVER be kept in your house! Readily available sweets are too tempting and too easy to get to. Example: You are sitting at home, it's 9:00 pm and you see a commercial for ice cream. Now you want some. If there is ice cream in your freezer, it's very easy to walk to the kitchen and get some so you probably will. However, if you have to get your shoes on, get in the car and drive to the store to get some, you probably won't.

Even if you have tremendous willpower 25 days out of the month and can walk by a fully stocked sweet cabinet in your house with no problem, there are going to be those days when things like stress, hormones, and emotions are going to kick in and give your willpower a run for its money. Don't take the chance. Get it out of your house!

*Eating Instinct #12: *Sleep your way to a leaner body!* **Do your best to get 7-8 hours sleep a night.**

Sleep! Glorious sleep! It's so important to our overall well-being including our stress level, immune system, attitude and efficiency. Getting 7-8 hours a night is important for each and every person. If you are one of those people thinking you get by just fine on 5-6 hours or less you are wrong. The truth is you have just *conditioned* yourself into believing you only need limited sleep. You are s*urviving* on less sleep but are you *thriving?* The answer is a big NO. Sleep is not just important it's critical. Scientists are now discovering that sleep deprivation contributes to depression, diabetes, heart disease and obesity. How exactly does sleep deprivation contribute to obesity? In a University of Chicago study researchers restricted a group of individuals to only 4 hours of sleep a night. After just 2 nights of sleep deprivation the individuals had an 18% decrease in the hormone Leptin which tells your brain when you are full and a 28% increase in the hormone Ghrelin which triggers hunger. Study after study back up this research. These same hormones were negatively affected with people getting 6 hours of sleep which many consider a full nights rest! How are you supposed to control your appetite when your hormones are driving you to eat more and not letting you know when you are full? No one has the tremendous willpower it would take to override these hormones day after day.

You have no choice. If you want to be lean and healthy, your body needs 7 to 8 hours of sleep every night.

*<u>Eating Instinct #13:</u> *Getting more than you bargained for with supplements?* **Take one brand name multiple vitamin daily such as Centrum or One a Day.**

Supplements are a multi-billion dollar industry. If you've been inside any health food store lately you may have noticed that the store is full of bottles of pills, powders, capsules and oils promising a healthier happier you. Do these pills and powders really deliver what they say or could they possibly do more harm than good?

Here's the deal: NO ONE is checking up on supplements. Supplement makers are accountable to NO ONE. There is absolutely NO government agency checking to see if what the manufacturers claim is in their product is actually in there. There is also NO ONE checking to see if there is anything in there that is *not* supposed to be in there such as contaminants. The FDA is only allowed to get involved when people are getting sick or injured due to supplements and complaints are filed with the FDA. The manufacturers are not even responsible for reporting any known injuries or illnesses involving their product! Hard to believe? Well it's true. In fact the following statement is directly from the FDA themselves:

By law (DSHEA), the manufacturer is responsible for ensuring that its dietary supplement products are safe before they are marketed. Unlike drug products that must be proven safe and effective for their intended use before marketing, there are no provisions in the law for FDA to "approve" dietary supplements for safety or effectiveness before they reach the consumer. Also unlike drug products, manufacturers and distributors of dietary supplements are not currently required by law to record, investigate or forward to the FDA any reports they receive of injuries or illnesses that may be related to the use of their products. Under DSHEA, once the product is marketed, FDA has the responsibility for showing that a dietary supplement is "unsafe," before it can take action to restrict the product's use or removal from the marketplace.

The only people doing any checking at all are a handful of consumer advocacy groups such as Consumerlabs.com. I am a huge fan of Consumerlabs.com. Their mission: *To identify the best quality health and nutritional products through independent testing.* They then share this information on their website and also share their findings with national news organizations such as MSNBC and CNN who routinely report on these findings.

Some of their findings are exactly what you might expect: some supplements don't have as much of an ingredient as they claim to have. However, what is even scarier is that sometimes supplements contain toxic levels of an ingredient or even contaminants such as lead!!! Here are just some of their recent findings:

- Some of the most popular supplements including resveratrol, probiotics, calcium supplements and Omega 3 fish oils were found to contain far less ingredient than what the label claims. Or in the case of vitamin A some manufacturers are claiming their product is the more desirable natural form of vitamin A when they actually contain the synthetic vitamin A.
- A popular womens multivitamin contained only 54% of the calcium stated on the label but even worse it contained 15.3 micrograms of lead per two tablet daily serving!
- One popular childrens multivitamin had substantially more vitamin A than stated on the label. In fact this product delivered 5400 units in a daily serving which is far above the tolerable level set for children. Vitamin A is a

fat soluble vitamin which means excess is not just passed through when we urinate like water soluble vitamins, but stored in our body fat and can build up to toxic levels in our bodies becoming potentially dangerous.

- 20% of arthritis supplements selected for testing were found to be contaminated or mislabeled.

To find out the names of these and other brands that have tested to be untrue to their labels you can visit www.consumberlabs.com yourself! See how your vitamins and supplements check out. They also have an extensive listing of FDA recalls and warnings on supplements that have made consumers sick.

Maybe your supplements check out just fine. Do you still want to be putting all that "stuff" in your system? Vitamins, minerals and herbs are in almost everyones homes these days. People are dumping all kinds of stuff into their bodies without giving it a second thought. We are trying to get health out of a bottle when true health comes from the food we put inside our bodies.

All it takes is one study suggesting that a particular vitamin or mineral is going to help you lose weight or be healthier and that supplement starts flying off the shelves! Let's take calcium for example. Everyone knows that you need calcium for strong bones. Many women I run into are taking calcium supplements. Some are taking very high doses. What's wrong with that? Well, first of all it does you no good to just swallow a bunch of calcium supplements if you aren't going to exercise. Exercise is the catalyst to get the calcium INTO your bones. Also, not all calcium can be utilized by your body and some is utilized more readily than others. Where does all that unutilized calcium go? Some studies have shown men who take in very high amounts of calcium have an increased risk of dying from prostate cancer. Other studies suggest women who ingest high doses of calcium might have more heart disease and may have a slightly increased risk of ovarian cancer. Some scientists are now suggesting that excessive calcium can damage arteries. The incidence of kidney stones has been on the rise since the calcium frenzy. Are they related? Some doctors think so.

Remember, just because a little is good doesn't mean a lot is better. Here is another example:

- Mega doses of vitamin C supplements can cause nausea, diarrhea, kidney stones and inflammation of the stomach lining (gastritis). Rarely, too much vitamin C can cause faintness, dizziness and fatigue. (Mayo clinic)

Another disturbing trend is people taking many different supplements to supposedly boost their immune systems so they don't end up on antibiotics. Why are they so afraid of antibiotics which are given under the advice of a physician and controlled by the FDA but perfectly comfortable with dumping tons of unproven unregulated supplements into their bodies???

Want to boost your immune system? Eat more fruits and vegetables, get more sleep, and drink more water.

My philosophy on supplements is simply this: I have a very strong theory that if you are deficient in a vitamin, your body may cause you to eat more food in search of the vitamin you are lacking in. Taking in extra calories you don't need, you may overeat and still not get the vitamin your body is searching for. What should you do to avoid this potential problem? Take one multivitamin a day and think of it as a "safety net". In case you miss out on a particular vitamin that day you are covered. Start by sticking with a big brand name multi such as Centrum or One a Day (or Flintstones for your kids)! Time and time again, these well-known brands are tested and deliver exactly what they say they do. They know they will be tested more frequently and they have a long running reputation to uphold so they make sure they get it right.

Unless you have been instructed otherwise by your personal physician, stick with the daily multi-vitamin. Yes, it's important to get your vitamins and minerals but get the majority of them through eating healthy whole foods! The way nature intended!

BODYINSTINCT "6 WEEK TOTAL TRANSFORMATION PROGRAM"

WEEK 4
FITNESS GUIDELINES:

<u>**Weight/resistance training program**</u>: Do some type of resistance training such as Hard-Body Yoga™, pilates or weightlifting for 30-60 minutes twice a week.

<u>**Cardio program**</u>: Three 20-minute cardio workouts a week done very intensely in an interval fashion. 4 minutes at or above your 75% range and the 5th minute at full blast then repeat this 4 times total to complete 20 minutes. Warm up and cool down do not count towards the 20 minutes. A heart rate monitor is highly recommended to make sure you are burning fat most efficiently. (to find your 75% range: 220 – your age x 75%) Do your cardio first thing in the morning on an empty stomach or immediately after your weight/resistance workout. Whenever possible, wait one hour after cardio before eating. **Add more intervals.**

NUTRITION PROGRAM EATING INSTINCTS:

- <u>**Eating Instinct #1:**</u> Eat unprocessed foods whenever possible (food in its natural state). Your diet should consist mainly of lean high quality protein, fruits & vegetables.
- <u>**Eating Instinct #2:**</u> Be a daytime eater. Always eat breakfast, make lunch your main meal, and think of dinner as a small light meal consisting of lean protein and vegetables.
- <u>**Eating Instinct #3:**</u> NEVER let more than 3 hours go by without food. Eat several small meals instead of 2-3 big

ones or supplement 3 regular meals with healthy unprocessed snacks such as fruit, veggies or nuts in between.

- **Eating Instinct #4:** Avoid most saturated fat and **all** hydrogenated oils (trans fats). The fat in your diet should be coming mostly from nuts, seeds, olives, and avocados. (oils should be used sparingly and should be cold or expeller pressed) Remove all products with hydrogenated or partially hydrogenated oils from your home.
- **Eating Instinct #5:** Drink at least **96** oz (12 cups) of water every day.
- **Eating Instinct #6:** Make sure you are getting lean high quality protein at least 3 times a day.
- **Eating Instinct #7:** Avoid eating after 7:00 pm or 12 hours after your regular wake up time.
- **Eating Instinct #8:** Restrict energy foods: nuts & seeds, fruit and especially starchy carbs (rice, pasta, bread, sugar, potatoes, and flour products) after 3:00 pm. You are what you eat after 3:00 pm!
- **Eating Instinct #9:** Limit alcohol intake to no more than 1 glass of wine or beer a day. (7 glasses a week)
- **Eating Instinct #10:** Don't drink your calories! This includes fruit & vegetable juices. Eat the whole fruit or vegetable instead!
- **Eating Instinct #11:** Restrict refined sugars and sweet snacks. (if desired you may have ONE small sweet snack per day before 3:00 pm) Do not keep ANY sweets in your house
- **Eating Instinct #12:** Do your best to get 7-8 hours sleep a night
- **Eating Instinct #13:** Take one brand name multiple vitamin daily such as Centrum or One a Day.
- **Eating Instinct #14: Eliminate all artificial sweeteners, colors and flavors.**
- **Eating Instinct #15: Restrict dairy products to no more than one 8 ounce serving per day. (Should be low fat)**

CHAPTER FOUR

PUTTING YOUR INSTINCTS TO THE TEST!

WEEK FOUR:

FITNESS GUIDELINES:

Shake your cardio up a little!

Strength and Resistance program: Remains the same

Cardio program: Add more intervals.

It is a great time to start having fun and playing around a little bit with your cardio by adding more intervals. Try 8 total intervals per 20 minute session instead of 4 or maybe do shorter intervals for 30 seconds more frequently. Or mix up shorter and longer intervals. It's good to change it a little bit every time or at least now and then. It's also a good idea to change what you do *for* your interval. For example, if you have been walking on a tread-mill and have been speeding up for your intervals try increasing the incline instead or a little bit of both. If you have been walking or running outside and using faster runs or sprints as your interval, try stepping up and down on a curb for a minute or doing some jumping jacks instead. Just play with it and keep it interesting!

WEEK FOUR ADDITIONAL EATING INSTINCTS:

*Note: water intake increases to 96 oz. (12 cups) a day

*<u>Eating Instinct #14</u>: *Get the yuck out!* **Eliminate all artificial sweeteners, colors and flavors.**

Artificial is the exact opposite of natural. I don't trust, and nor should you, man-made ingredients not found in nature. Manufacturers of these artificial ingredients will tell you they are safe and so will some government agencies like the FDA. Sometimes they will declare them safe, change their minds, and then change their minds back again. The FDA originally approved the artificial sweetener saccharin, then tried to get it banned but was only granted a warning label, then removed the warning label. So which is it? Safe or unsafe?

Speaking of the FDA, did you know there is an actual page on the FDA's website entitled EAFUS which stands for "everything added to food in the United States"? I find that rather comical. I can just see a bunch of government bigwigs sitting around deciding what to call a webpage that lists over 2000 food additives in our food including preservatives, colors, flavors, sweeteners etc... Gee let's just call it "everything added to food in the United States".

How about the hydrogenated oil (trans fat) issue? Chemists started messing around with the hydrogen atoms in good fats and declared that they had increased shelf life in products and that this new altered fat was perfectly healthy. They went so far as to claim that Margarine (a tub of trans fat) is better for you than butter!! – fast forward a few decades and many heart attacks later, and we are now told by the USDA and the FDA that trans fatty acids (aka hydrogenated oils) are extremely unhealthy and should be avoided completely.

These examples and many others just like them do not increase my confidence in statements by any government agency that artificial colors, flavors, and sweeteners are safe.

Let's start with artificial sweeteners: Many studies of these sweeteners claim they are safe. Other studies claim exactly the opposite. Regardless of whether or not they are good for you, the question remains are they doing you any good in maintaining a leaner body? The overwhelming answer is no.
Look at what these findings suggest from an 8 year study at the University Of Texas Health Science Center:

- People who drank diet soft drinks don't lose weight. In fact, they gain weight
- For *each* can of diet soft drink consumed each day, a person's risk of obesity went up 41%

Now check out these findings from a recent Purdue University study:
- consuming a food sweetened with no-calorie saccharin can lead to greater bodyweight gain and adiposity (fat) than would consuming the same food sweetened with high-calorie sugar.

Boston University School of medicine researchers came to the following conclusions:

- adults who drink one or more diet sodas a day have about a 50% higher risk of "metabolic syndrome" – a set of risk factors that include excessive fat around the waist, low levels of "good" cholesterol, and high blood pressure to name a few.

How can this be? Aren't all of these artificially sweetened food and drinks supposed to help us lose weight? Why would you gain weight from diet drinks and food? Here are some possible answers:

1. When your body tastes the sweet taste of artificial sweeteners it expects a certain number of calories to go with that taste. When it doesn't get them it goes in search of those calories promised and not delivered, causing an individual to consume excess calories.
2. The sweetness of diet soda causes an individual to develop a preference for sweet foods.

It could be answer number 1 or 2 or a combination of both. Regardless, artificial sweeteners are not doing you any good and may be harmful to your body.

Artificial colors have their own cause for concern. Just the fact that most artificial colors are derived from coal and petroleum should raise eyebrows. Others such as carmine are derived from insects. Carmine provides color in the red, pink and purple range and is obtained from female cochineal beetles. Yuck. Artificial colors are used mainly in foods with low nutritive values to make them more appealing especially to children. They are mostly found in high sugar cereals, candies, sodas and snacks: foods you should generally be staying away from by now anyway. Consumer advocacy groups such as the "Center for Science in the Public Interest" have been at the FDA for years to ban the use of many artificial colors claiming they cause hyperactivity in children and have been linked to certain cancers. One thing is for certain; they are definitely NOT contributing anything healthy to your diet and are more likely doing harm.

Artificial flavors are mostly chemical compounds that are produced to mimic the taste of natural flavors. As in all aspects of food and nutrition, the natural choice is always a better one. The recent news about factory workers dying of lung disease in food flavoring plants that were producing artificial butter flavor is alarming. The disease is also known as popcorn workers lung because of its prevalence in factories producing microwave popcorn flavored with the artificial butter flavor. In only 5 years over $100 million dollars has been paid out by flavoring manufacturers in lawsuits brought by workers with popcorn workers lung. Must be something to it. I would like to know is it just breathing in the stuff that may kill you or might eating it not be such a good idea also? I say we don't eat it or inhale it! And that goes for all other artificial flavors too!

*Eating Instinct #15: *Is milk only for baby cows?* **Restrict dairy products to no more than one 8 ounce serving per day. (Should be low fat)**

Let's get one thing straight: Dairy and dairy products are NOT necessary for human beings. We are the only species that drinks milk from another species. A human drinking cows milk is about as natural as a dog drinking zebra milk.

Here is a little back up information:

Over 30 million Americans are "lactose intolerant" or lacking the enzyme needed to digest milk. Although most everyone has the milk digesting enzyme (lactase) as a baby, most bodies naturally stop producing it around the age of 2 when a child would normally be weaned. It is NOT normal for the body to make lactase after early childhood. In fact, the "lactose intolerant" people are the ones whose bodies are getting it right! The rest of us have digestive systems that have been conditioned to ignore the bodies' natural instincts to stop drinking milk after weaning. These "milk friendly" bodies have ancestral backgrounds rooted mainly in Northern and Western Europe where there is a long strong history of dairy farming. Because of the prevalence of dairy in these areas through the centuries, these bodies have encouraged and conditioned themselves to continue to produce lactase long after nature would normally stop.

In other words, the high numbers of lactose intolerant individuals are trying to tell us something: YOU DON'T NEED AND SHOULDN'T BE DRINKING MILK!!!

Other reasons to not drink milk:

- several studies have shown a link between the early introduction of cow's milk in an infant's diet and type 1 diabetes.
- Milk isn't the only or even best source of calcium. Other calcium rich foods include leafy greens, baked beans and broccoli. The calcium in these foods also has a higher bioavailability than the calcium in milk which means it is better utilized in the body.
- High intake of dairy increases the risk of prostate cancer and possibly ovarian cancer.
- Casein (a major protein found in milk) can be difficult to digest for many individuals and is strongly linked to chronic ear infections, sinus congestion, acne and eczema.

Believe it or not, as much as we don't NEED dairy, I do believe it has a place in our diet.

The Harvard School of Medicine recently suggested no more than 1 or 2 servings of Dairy a day which has always been my recommendation as well. I also highly recommend those choices be in the form of yogurt or cheese instead of milk. Yogurt and cheese are a more preferred and easier digested source of dairy. They have much less lactose than milk and contain probiotics. Probiotics are live microorganisms in fermented foods. Their potential benefits include the prevention of colon cancer, lower cholesterol, lower blood pressure, improved immune functions, prevention of infections, reduced inflammation, improvement of mineral absorption and a decrease in antibiotic associated diarrhea.

Low fat cheeses and yogurts are a better choice than *fat free*. I have never been a fan of "fat free" products as they are usually pumped up with a bunch of junk like sugar, white flour and other fillers to replace the fat. You also *need* some of the fat that naturally occurs in dairy products to slow down the digestion of the dairy giving your body more time to fully digest the casein protein therefore reducing the previously mentioned side effects from undigested casein.

I would also HIGHLY recommend buying organic or "hormone free" dairy products. Dairy cows are treated with growth hormones to make them mature faster and to produce more milk. In fact they are forced to produce about 10 times more milk a day than they normally would to feed their young.

They are also administered antibiotics regularly to keep them disease free as they are warehoused in huge overcrowded sheds and treated like milk machines and often develop mastitis (infection of the mammary glands).

Where do you think those antibiotics and growth hormones (aka steroids) end up? Yes! In their milk! If you or someone you know has ever breastfed you are probably aware that there are very strict guidelines as to what drugs a mother may take while nursing. In fact the majority of drugs are **not** recommended for nursing mothers. The reason is the drugs end up concentrating in the breast milk and are passed on to the baby in quantities that could be detrimental to the Childs health. Well, in the case of dairy, think of the cow as your mother on large doses of steroids and antibiotics and **you** are the nursing baby. Yuck!

Milk produced organically is from cows not treated with antibiotics or steroids. There are also some dairy products that are not organic but are from cows not treated with growth hormones. Personally I would like to avoid both hormones and antibiotics but the more potentially dangerous of the two is definitely the growth hormones. It's important to realize that growth hormones encourage everything to grow in your body – good and bad. Imagine if you have a small precancerous or cancerous growth somewhere in your body. Do you want to possibly encourage that growth by consuming dairy products with high levels of growth hormone on a daily basis? Another case for avoiding dairy with growth hormone is the fact that our children in this country are going through puberty earlier and earlier and that has been strongly linked to the amount of growth hormones in our food!

The Reason to avoid the antibiotics in milk is obvious. Why would you want to put unnecessary antibiotics in your body every day of your life? This is harmful to our immune system and helps to develop antibiotic resistance and the emergence of antibiotic resistant "suberbugs" such as Mrsa.

To sum this one up: Keep dairy intake low and whenever possible choose organic dairy products.

THE WEEK FOUR SELF-TEST

Ok, by now you should be quite comfortable with the "you are what you eat after 3 pm" instinct. Your body should have adjusted and is now used to eating only repair and recovery foods (protein and vegetables) after 3 pm and eliminating energy foods. Just to be sure you are on track there is a very simple and easy self-test you can do. Choose one day this week and stop eating at 3 pm. Have your breakfast, your first snack, your lunch, and then your second snack as close to 3 pm as possible and that's it. You can keep drinking your water all day. Most everyone's reaction to this information is a gasp! Don't be so dramatic. Seriously, if you were having outpatient surgery or a medical procedure and your doctor asked you to not eat after 3 pm the day before, you would think nothing of it and just do it. That's exactly the attitude you should take with this. If you have been doing everything correctly most of the time and have become a "daytime eater" eating the majority of your calories early in the day then this should be a walk in the park for you.

You can do this by looking ahead at your schedule for the week and choosing a day that you think would be good for you to give the self-test a try OR you can just wing it one day. A lot of people choose to wing it because they find themselves in a day that just seems conducive to not eating after 3 pm.

How do you know if you passed the test? That's easy. If you feel like you would have liked to eat but it's no big deal that you didn't then you passed. If you start to experience one of the following reactions:

Lightheadedness
Irritability
Extreme hunger
Shakiness

You did not pass and you need to eat something right away. Don't beat yourself up if you did not pass the self-test. I would suggest you just take a good look at your daily food intake after 3 pm and make the necessary adjustments to insure you are eating only lean protein and vegetables after 3 pm and in smaller amounts. I would also suggest you do week 4 for 2 weeks and try the self-test again before moving onto week 5. Remember that this is not a race but a program designed to get you back to your natural eating instincts and not everyone has to be on the exact same timeline. If you want to do every week for two weeks and take 12 weeks to go through the program then so be it! It's all good!

If you did pass the self-test with no problem than congratulations! You are exactly where you need to be to move on to week 5 and you have become a successful daytime eater frontloading your calories and eating for your energy expenditure! You are eating *with* instead of against your circadian rhythm!

BODYINSTINCT "6 WEEK TOTAL TRANSFORMATION PROGRAM"

WEEK 5
FITNESS GUIDELINES:

<u>**Weight/resistance training program**</u>: Do some type of resistance training such as Hard-Body Yoga™, Pilates or weightlifting for 30-60 minutes twice a week.

<u>**Cardio program**</u>: Three 20-minute cardio workouts a week done very intensely in an interval fashion. 4 minutes at or above your 75% range and the 5th minute at full blast then repeat this 4 times total to complete 20 minutes.   A heart rate monitor is highly recommended to make sure you are burning fat most efficiently. (to find your 75% range: 220 – your age x 75%) Do your cardio first thing in the morning on an empty stomach or immediately after your weight/resistance workout. Whenever possible, wait one hour after cardio before eating.

NUTRITION PROGRAM EATING INSTINCTS:

- <u>**Eating Instinct #1:**</u> Eat unprocessed foods whenever possible (food in its natural state). Your diet should consist mainly of lean high quality protein, fruits & vegetables.
- <u>**Eating Instinct #2:**</u> Be a daytime eater. Always eat breakfast, make lunch your main meal, and think of dinner as a small light meal consisting of lean protein and vegetables.

- **Eating Instinct #3:** NEVER let more than 3 hours go by without food. Eat several small meals instead of 2-3 big ones or supplement 3 regular meals with healthy unprocessed snacks such as fruit, veggies or nuts in between.
- **Eating Instinct #4:** Avoid most saturated fat and **all** hydrogenated oils (trans fats). The fat in your diet should be coming mostly from nuts, seeds, olives, and avocados. (oils should be used sparingly and should be cold or expeller pressed) Remove all products with hydrogenated or partially hydrogenated oils from your home.
- **Eating Instinct #5:** Drink at least **112 oz. (14 cups)** of water ever day.
- **Eating Instinct #6:** Make sure you are getting lean high quality protein at least 3 times a day.
- **Eating Instinct #7:** Avoid eating after 7:00 pm or 12 hours after your regular wake up time.
- **Eating Instinct #8:** Restrict energy foods: nuts & seeds, fruit and especially starchy carbs (rice, pasta, bread, sugar, potatoes, and flour products) after 3:00 pm. You are what you eat after 3:00 pm!
- **Eating Instinct #9:** Limit alcohol intake to no more than 1 glass of wine or beer a day. (7 glasses a week)
- **Eating Instinct #10:** Don't drink your calories! This includes fruit & vegetable juices. Eat the whole fruit or vegetable instead!
- **Eating Instinct #11:** Restrict refined sugars and sweet snacks. (if desired you may have ONE small sweet snack per day before 3:00 pm) Do not keep ANY sweets in your house
- **Eating Instinct #12:** Do your best to get 7-8 hours sleep a night.
- **Eating Instinct #13:** Take one brand name multiple vitamin daily such as Centrum or One a Day.

- **<u>Eating Instinct #14:</u>** Eliminate all artificial sweeteners, colors and flavors.
- **<u>Eating Instinct #15:</u>** Restrict dairy products to no more than one 8 ounce serving per day. (should be low fat)
- **<u>Eating Instinct #16:</u> Restrict caffeine to no more than two 8 oz. cups a day. Tea or coffee.**

CHAPTER FIVE

A LITTLE EXTRA BOOST!

FITNESS GUIDELINES:

Cardio and weight resistance programs remain the same.

WEEK FIVE ADDITONAL EATING INSTINCTS:

***Note: Water intake increases to 112 oz. (14 cups) a day.**

*<u>**Eating Instinct #16:**</u> *Caffeine: Friend or foe?* **Restrict caffeine to no more than two 8 oz. cups a day. Tea or coffee.**

A cup of joe can make you feel energized but, is it bad for you? Or could it possibly even make you a healthier person? In the past, coffee drinking had a kind of stigma about it. Many people thought it would improve your health to stop consuming coffee or it would at least be better to switch to tea. Studies were done that concluded coffee drinking was detrimental to your health. Now we know that just isn't so. Better conducted larger more recent studies on humans have shown *increased* health benefits from coffee in many areas. In fact latest research suggests that coffee may protect against type 2 diabetes, Parkinson's disease, colon cancer, cirrhosis of the liver and possibly even heart disease!

Although researchers believe the caffeine in coffee is responsible for most of these desired health effects there are also many other healthy compounds in coffee such as powerful flavanoids and antioxidants that become even more potent during the roasting process.

Tea has health benefits as well but surprisingly the research on the health benefits of tea is not as promising as that on coffee. Possibly because tea is not as high in caffeine as coffee and the caffeine is contributing highly to the health benefits. There are many antioxidants in tea (especially in green tea which has not been fermented like other teas) that have shown benefits in fighting certain types of cancer and heart disease however these are only laboratory tests and researchers have been unsuccessful in replicating these results in tests on actual humans.

Any cons with coffee or tea? Well, there are components in coffee that have been shown to raise cholesterol but by drinking filtered coffee you eliminate these substances. They remain behind in the filter. Then there is the modest increase in osteoporosis in women under 65 who are heavy coffee drinkers (4 cups or more a day) and have inadequate amounts of calcium in their diet. Coffee and tea can also cause heartburn and mess around with your sleep if you drink them too late in the day. Keep in mind that coffee and tea are mild diuretics which increase urine secretion but that is easily remedied by drinking enough water which you certainly are on week 5!

Since there is little evidence of health risks and some strong evidence of health benefits I say if you are already a tea or coffee drinker then go ahead and enjoy your tea or coffee. By now you know the BodyInstinct theme that if a little is good for you then a lot is NOT necessarily better so as with most everything else I recommend moderation. Limiting your caffeine consumption to two 8 oz cups a day is a good idea. Be it tea or coffee. It is also best for you to drink coffee or tea without milk, sugar, creamers or artificial sweeteners. In fact these additives could possible negate some of the health benefits of tea and coffee.

One more suggestion when it comes to caffeine. One of the best times to consume caffeine is immediately before your 20 minute cardio workout. Studies have shown that ingesting a cup of black coffee or plain tea before doing your cardio increases fat burning by triggering the release of more fatty acids to be burned up as fuel. I can personally tell you that I can almost instinctually *feel* my body burning more fat when I consume caffeine before a cardio workout. The stimulating effect of the caffeine also increases exercise performance and that may be a contributing factor as well. Remember that it has to be plain coffee or tea with absolutely NOTHING in it whatsoever so that you are still exercising on an empty calorie free stomach. If that's a little too hardcore for you than simply don't do it. It's not near as influential in burning fat as is working out first thing in the morning on an empty stomach, but it definitely is an extra push for your body to burn fat.

BODYINSTINCT "6 WEEK TOTAL TRANSFORMATION PROGRAM"

WEEK 6
FITNESS GUIDELINES:

<u>**Weight/resistance training program**</u>: Do some type of resistance training such as Hard-Body Yoga™, Pilates or weightlifting for 30-60 minutes twice a week.

<u>**Cardio program**</u>: Three 20-minute cardio workouts a week done very intensely in an interval fashion. 4 minutes at or above your 75% range and the 5th minute at full blast then repeat this 4 times total to complete 20 minutes. A heart rate monitor is highly recommended to make sure you are burning fat most efficiently. (to find your 75% range: 220 – your age x 75%) Do your cardio first thing in the morning on an empty stomach or immediately after your weight/resistance workout. Whenever possible, wait one hour after cardio before eating.

NUTRITION PROGRAM EATING INSTINCTS:

- <u>**Eating Instinct #1:**</u> Eat unprocessed foods whenever possible (food in its natural state). Your diet should consist mainly of lean high quality protein, fruits & vegetables.
- <u>**Eating Instinct #2:**</u> Be a daytime eater. Always eat breakfast, make lunch your main meal, and think of dinner as a small light meal consisting of lean protein and vegetables.
- <u>**Eating Instinct #3:**</u> NEVER let more than 3 hours go by without food. Eat several small meals instead of 2-3 big

ones or supplement 3 regular meals with healthy unprocessed snacks such as fruit, veggies or nuts in between.

- **Eating Instinct #4:** Avoid most saturated fat and **all** hydrogenated oils (trans fats). The fat in your diet should be coming mostly from nuts, seeds, olives, and avocados. (oils should be used sparingly and should be cold or expeller pressed) Remove all products with hydrogenated or partially hydrogenated oils from your home.
- **Eating Instinct #5:** Drink at least **120 oz. (16 cups)** of water ever day.
- **Eating Instinct #6:** Make sure you are getting lean high quality protein at least 3 times a day.
- **Eating Instinct #7:** Avoid eating after 7:00 pm or 12 hours after your regular wake up time.
- **Eating Instinct #8:** Restrict energy foods: nuts & seeds, fruit and especially starchy carbs (rice, pasta, bread, sugar, potatoes, and flour products) after 3:00 pm. You are what you eat after 3:00 pm!
- **Eating Instinct #9:** Limit alcohol intake to no more than 1 glass of wine or beer a day. (7 glasses a week)
- **Eating Instinct #10:** Don't drink your calories! This includes fruit & vegetable juices. Eat the whole fruit or vegetable instead!
- **Eating Instinct #11:** Restrict refined sugars and sweet snacks. (if desired you may have ONE small sweet snack per day before 3:00 pm) Do not keep ANY sweets in your house
- **Eating Instinct #12:** Do your best to get 7-8 hours sleep a night.
- **Eating Instinct #13:** Take one brand name multiple vitamin daily such as Centrum or One a Day.
- **Eating Instinct #14:** Eliminate all artificial sweeteners, colors and flavors.

- **Eating Instinct #15:** Restrict dairy products to no more than one 8 ounce serving per day. (should be low fat)
- **Eating Instinct #16:** Restrict caffeine to no more than two 8 oz. cups a day. Tea or coffee.

CHAPTER SIX

TIGHTENING UP FOR A WEEK!

WEEK SIX

FITNESS GUIDELINES:

Cardio and weight resistance programs remain the same.

WEEK SIX ADDITIONAL EATING INSTINCTS:

*Note: Water intake increases to 120 oz. (16 cups) a day.

Except for the additional water intake (are your back teeth float-
ing yet?) there are no additional fitness guidelines or eating instincts for week 6. If you aren't already, this would be the week to
take each and every fitness guideline and eating instinct from all
the previous weeks and put them into full force.

BODYINSTINCT "6 WEEK TOTAL TRANSFORMATION PROGRAM"

ONGOING PROGRAM FITNESS GUIDELINES:

<u>Weight/resistance training program</u>: Do some type of resistance training such as Hard-Body Yoga™, Pilates or weightlifting for 30-60 minutes twice a week. **After 6 weeks of training, take the seventh week off to avoid overuse injuries and burnout. Do active rest.**

<u>Cardio program</u>: Three 20-minute cardio workouts a week done very intensely in an interval fashion. 4 minutes at or above your 75% range and the 5th minute at full blast then repeat this 4 times total to complete 20 minutes. Warm up and cool down do not count towards the 20 minutes. A heart rate monitor is highly recommended to make sure you are in your range and burning fat most efficiently. (to find your 75% range: 220 – your age x 75%) Do your cardio first thing in the morning on an empty stomach or immediately after your resistance workout. Wait one hour after cardio before eating. **After 6 weeks of training, take the seventh week off to avoid overuse injuries and burnout. Do active rest.**

NUTRITION PROGRAM EATING INSTINCTS:

- **<u>Eating Instinct #1</u>:** Eat unprocessed foods whenever possible (food in its natural state). Your diet should consist mainly of lean high quality protein, fruits & vegetables.

121

- **Eating Instinct #2:** Be a daytime eater. Always eat breakfast, make lunch your main meal, and think of dinner as a small light meal consisting of lean protein and vegetables.
- **Eating Instinct #3:** NEVER let more than 3 hours go by without food. Eat several small meals instead of 2-3 big ones or supplement 3 regular meals with healthy unprocessed snacks such as fruit, veggies or nuts in between.
- **Eating Instinct #4:** Avoid most saturated fat and **all** hydrogenated oils (trans fats). The fat in your diet should be coming mostly from nuts, seeds, olives, and avocados. (oils should be used sparingly and should be cold or expeller pressed) Remove all products with hydrogenated or partially hydrogenated oils from your home.
- **Eating Instinct #5: Drink only water and stay hydrated. Avoid waiting until you become thirsty.**
- **Eating Instinct #6:** Make sure you are getting lean high quality protein at least 3 times a day.
- **Eating Instinct #7:** Avoid eating after 7:00 pm or 12 hours after your regular wake up time.
- **Eating Instinct #8:** Restrict energy foods: nuts & seeds, fruit and especially starchy carbs (rice, pasta, bread, sugar, potatoes, and flour products) after 3:00 pm. You are what you eat after 3:00 pm!
- **Eating Instinct #9:** Limit alcohol intake to no more than 1 glass of wine or beer a day. (7 glasses a week)
- **Eating Instinct #10:** Don't drink your calories! This includes fruit & vegetable juices. Eat the whole fruit or vegetable instead!
- **Eating Instinct #11:** Restrict refined sugars and sweet snacks. (if desired you may have ONE small sweet snack per day before 3:00 pm) Do not keep ANY sweets in your house.
- **Eating Instinct #12:** Do your best to get 7-8 hours sleep a night.

- **Eating Instinct #13:** Take one brand name multiple vitamin daily such as Centrum or One a Day.
- **Eating Instinct #14:** Eliminate all artificial sweeteners, colors and flavors.
- **Eating Instinct #15:** Restrict dairy products to no more than one 8 ounce serving per day. (should be low fat)
- **Eating Instinct #16:** Restrict caffeine to no more than two 8 oz. cups a day. Tea or coffee.

CHAPTER SEVEN

THE ONGOING BODYINSTINCT LIFE PROGRAM:

A lifetime of good health and a lean strong body!

FITNESS GUIDELINES:

Enjoy a weeks rest! Your body and mind deserve it!

<u>Strength and Resistance program:</u> **After 6 weeks of training, take the seventh week off to avoid overuse injuries and burnout. Do active rest.**

<u>Cardio program:</u> **After 6 weeks of training, take the seventh week off to avoid overuse injuries and burnout. Do active rest.**

Yes! Rest! Just as important as exercise! Even though the BodyInstinct Program gets you maximum exercise results with minimum time invested (only 2 to 2½ hours a week) your body *and* mind still need extended periods of rest!

Eventually you will burn out or become injured if you don't periodically give your body a full weeks rest. Go through your calendar and draw a line through every seventh week and that's your week off (6 weeks on and one week off)! You may feel like you are on a roll and hesitate to take a week off but trust me on this one: Do it! It will be the best move you can make! It will give your body time to heal up any little overuse injuries that may be cropping up even though you don't feel them yet and maybe even more importantly it gives your brain something to look forward to!

On those days when you are not so enthused about getting on the treadmill or going outside for your run, take a look at your calendar and see when your next week off is. That will be enough to keep you going! Kind of like the light at the end of the 6 week tunnel! If you keep up with your eating instincts you will not gain any fat or lose any muscle on your week off. Promise! When you return to your program after your week off you will be stronger in the body and the mind. Your body will be rested and ready to roll and your brain will be begging for the endorphins it has been missing.

Don't take the rest week too literally and veg out on the couch for a week. Instead do "active rest". An example of active rest would be to go kayaking, go for a leisurely bike ride or a leisurely walk with your kids or dog, shoot some hoops or go play in the pool or ocean (not swim laps). I like to tell clients that to make sure you are not overdoing it the activity should be something you can do in flip flops or bare feet. The activity should also not get you winded or out of breath whatsoever.

ONGOING ADDITIONAL EATING INSTINCTS:

*Eating Instinct #5: Drink only water and stay hydrated. Avoid waiting until you become thirsty.

The only thing that changes in your eating instincts is you no longer need to monitor or measure the amount of water you drink! Just as with everything else once your instincts are uncovered, your body instinctually knows how much water and hydration you need on a day to day basis. After the past 6 weeks of drinking all the required water and getting your body used to what it feels like to be thoroughly hydrated your instincts will kick back in and ask for exactly what your body needs on a day to day basis. Different days require different amounts of water consumption. On days that you workout or the weather is hot and sunny or you eat a lot of salt your body will need and request more water than on days that are cooler or you are less active.

I still believe it is important to drink a big glass of water before sitting down to a meal so that you don't overeat in search of water in your food. I also think it's a good idea to have a water bottle available around you all day that you can sip off of so that you avoid waiting until you are overly thirsty to go look for water.

WHAT HAPPENS NOW???

By now your body should be very used to all the eating instincts. In fact they should be firing off by themselves like little internal reminders. Yeah, kind of like...........................your bodies natural instincts! And that's exactly what they are! Your bodies own natural inherent instincts uncovered and back at work! Remember they are reborn instincts! And just like a newborn they need to be paid attention to! The longer you pay attention to them the stronger they will become until it's an overwhelming force from within driving you to eat correctly along with your circadian rhythm!

It's important to know many of the people who have been through the BodyInstinct program have experienced an even bigger fat loss in the second six weeks following the ongoing life program. I am telling you this to encourage you to keep it up and you will continue to experience body fat loss for a long time to come! Remember! The BodyInstinct program is NOT some quick fix lose a lot now and gain it all back later program. BodyInstinct was designed to give you a permanent body fat loss of 1-2 pounds per week for as long as you want to keep losing!

This program takes 6 weeks to fully implement but is intended to be used for a lifetime! You will never have to feel that you are dieting again. You will only be allowing your natural instincts to take back over your body and give you new eating and thinking habits. The ideas presented to you in this program can be implemented anywhere, anytime. Any restaurant, vacation, family get together, party, or special occasion can still be enjoyed while using the program. The BodyInstinct Program will forever change the way you think about food and fitness. Change your thoughts, change your body, change your life!!!

BODYINSTINCT BOOSTERS: PUSHING PAST STICKING POINTS AND BALANCING OUT PERIODS OF LESS THAN IDEAL EATING.

The three following tools are for you to use to either push past a sticking point in your fat loss or balance out a day or more of eating out of whack. If it's pushing past a sticking point that you are trying to accomplish you won't stay stuck for long. If your eating has been out of whack with the BodyInstinct program NEVER let yourself feel guilty just choose one of the following three ways to balance out that day or more of out of whack eating. Creating balance is so much better than creating guilt.

1. First and foremost you can do the program at 100% for a week or more instead of between 80% and 100%. That will always be enough to keep burning the fat or balancing out the body. How do you make sure you are doing it 100%? Do all of the required fitness instincts exactly the way you are supposed to and follow the One Sheet BodyInstinct Structured Eating Plan to the T. Following The One Sheet BodyInstinct Structured Eating Plan *is* doing the program at 100%.

2. Once a week you can do the "self-test" and stop eating at 3 pm. If It's pretty much effortless, then you will know you are still on track and have not been eating too much later in the day. It will also be a little extra metabolism tweaker/fat burner. It's a great way to give yourself a little extra kick in the butt. In fact you can stop eating at 3 pm as many days of the week as you want and really speed up your progress or of course balance out any undesirable eating. I have clients who regularly stop eating after 3 pm a day or more every week. I will still occasionally use this as a balancing tool for a day or two at a time.

3. Do the BodyInstinct Cleanse. I personally despise most cleanses and detox's. Initially mostly water weight is lost, the fat loss is minimal and then you start breaking down muscle for fuel which as we know, slows down your metabolism and makes it easier than ever to gain weight when you go off the cleanse or detox. The BodyInstinct cleanse is more of a healthy whole food approach to cleansing the body. Nothing artificial or processed even in a small way. It's very doable in any environment you find yourself and you will not feel depleted, tired or deprived in any way and you will NOT lose muscle. The best part about it is you can do it for as little or as long as you want. Even doing the BodyInstinct cleanse for 1 day feels great and can get you back on track. Since it is not a deprivation cleanse you can do it indefinitely. You decide what you need to balance your body. Many of my clients like to do it for as much as a week or two after the holidays or after an extended vacation to balance out unhealthy eating. I myself will sometimes do it for one day to balance out a day that I may have done less than 80%. It's a great tool for creating balance.

BODYINSTINCT CLEANSE

Yes Anytime of day
All vegetables
Lean protein (meat, fish, chicken, pork)
Eggs
Yes before 3 pm only
Nuts & seeds (1 handful a day)
Oatmeal (breakfast only)
Beans (all kinds)
All fruit
Tea or coffee (reg and decaf) no more than 2-8 ounce cups per day plain

NO
Sugar
Bread or flour products
Rice
Potatoes
Pasta
Dairy products
Anything processed
No artificial sweeteners, colors, flavors

*drink 1 gallon of water each day
*balsamic or red wine vinegar on salads only
*dry spices only
*Certain foods should be organic please refer to the "dirty dozen" list at the end of chapter one
*If it's a food not mentioned on this list then it's a no.

All three ideas I mentioned can be used to balance out less than ideal eating. These tools are necessary to stop the "I blew it" syndrome. The "I blew it so badly this weekend that I feel I am back where I started so why bother". No you are not back where you started but you will be if you go with this guilty feeling. Instead shift your thinking to "so what if I ate whatever I wanted whenever I wanted this weekend, I can stop eating the next few days at 3 pm and completely void out the out of wack eating. Or I can do the BodyInstinct cleanse for a few days or get out my structured eating plan and follow it perfectly for the next few days or more. No need to jump ship! You have options and options that work!!

Since so much of health & fitness is mental an even better mental strategy for balancing is balancing BEFORE hand or being pro active. For instance if you have a vacation weekend coming up or have a big event that you know will be something that makes your eating "out of wack" to a degree, then for a few days BEFORE the event or weekend use one of the three tools! Now when the event or weekend is over you are right where you need to be and you don't even have to balance out because you pre-balanced! Just get back on track and you are good to go!

At the back of this book you will find The BodyInstinct Recipes. The BodyInstinct Recipes are from myself and also contributions from some of my clients. Give the ones that appeal to you a try. There are not tons of recipes just to fill up space but rather a few things that are tried and true and REALLY yummy and REALLY good for you! I love them all but the two that have EVERYONE won over are the BodyInstinct Banana Bread/Muffins and the BodyInstinct Corn and Bean Salsa!!! Both are always a big hit at parties and events and I am always asked for the recipe.

You are now independent but not completely on your own! It's important to know that you always have lots of references. This book for starters, my TariRose.com facebook page which you can follow for up to the minute new ideas and products to enhance your BodyInstinct Program and www.TariRose.com where you can register for email updates and I will also keep you posted on upcoming BodyInstinct webinars, BodyInstinct apps, new book and video releases and the latest health & fitness information available.

You now have the knowledge *and* the power!! The BodyInstinct Program has forever changed the way you will think about food and fitness. Change your thoughts, change your body, change your life!!!

BODYINSTINCT 6 WEEK PROGRAM BREAKFAST IDEAS AND RECIPES WWW.TARIROSE.COM

BodyInstinct pancakes:
1 cup Aunt Jemima Whole Wheat pancake mix
1 cup organic milk or soy or rice milk
1 egg
¼ cup ground flax meal

*combine all ingredients and cook as usual using nonstick cooking spray on pan
*may add blueberries, bananas, or other fruits if desired.
*Makes 6 pancakes (2 pancakes = 1 serving) extra pancakes freeze well and can be microwaved for breakfast another day

BodyInstinct shake:
Any 2 fruits or 2 cups of fruit
¼ cup of Fage lowfat yogurt or other brand of Greek lowfat yogurt
1 tblsp peanut butter or flax meal
If necessary, just enough water for desired consistency

*blend all ingredients in blender

BodyInstinct Oatmeal Cake:
4 egg whites
1 banana
½ cup oatmeal (old fashioned uncooked)
Nuts or peanut butter

*blend all ingredients in blender
*pour into microwave safe large cereal bowl sprayed with cooking spray
*microwave on high for 3–4 minutes depending on your microwave
*let cool slightly then turn bowl over and pop out cake.

BodyInstinct French Toast

4 slices of Marathon High Protein Bread or whole grain bread
2 eggs
¼ cup organic lowfat milk or soymilk
¼ tsp vanilla extract
1 tsp cinnamon

*mix all ingredients except bread in a bowl with wisk or fork until foamy
*soak each piece of bread well in the mixture and place on pre-heated frying pan that has been coated with cooking spray.
*flip and cook both sides of bread until light brown
*serve with small amount of all natural maple syrup and berries if desired
*2 slices = 1 serving. Additional slices can be frozen and micro-waved for breakfast another day.

BodyInstinct Banana Bread/Muffins

¼ cup of butter softened
¼ cup ground flax meal
½ cup sugar
2 large eggs
1 ½ cups of whole wheat flour
1 teaspoon baking soda
1 teaspoon salt
4 very ripe bananas mashed

½ cup of Fage 2% yogurt
1 teaspoon vanilla
½ cup chopped walnuts or pecans (if desired)

*preheat oven to 350
*lightly butter or pan spray pan
*Blend or mix all ingredients together
*pour into prepared pan
Use the following baking times:
One large loaf pan = 45 minutes
One 12 count muffin pan = 20 minutes
Four small loaf pans = 25 minutes
Bake until toothpick inserted in center comes out clean
*can also be enjoyed as a snack and can also be frozen to be enjoyed later

BODYINSTINCT 6 WEEK PROGRAM DINNER IDEAS AND RECIPES WWW.TARIROSE.COM

BodyInstinct Pork chops & Zucchini

Boneless lean pork chops
Greek seasoning (available in most all grocery stores)
2 large zucchini
1 small onion
Grated parmesan
Olive oil

*Lightly coat pork chops with Greek seasoning. Coat a grill pan with cooking spray and heat to med high. Put chops in pan for one minute on each side to sear then turn pan down to medium and cook until done.
*slice zucchini and onion very thin and spread in small glass baking pan. Drizzle lightly with olive oil and sprinkle lightly with parmesan cheese. Cover cook on high in microwave for 10 minutes.

BodyInstinct Main Meal Salad

One bag of organic pre-washed lettuce of your choice
½ cup of organic lowfat provolone or mild white cheddar cheese cubed organic or hormone free
2 or 3 slices of lean prosciutto ham torn into small strips
½ pound of cooked and shelled medium shrimp cut into 2 or 3 pieces each
1 cup of cherry tomatoes
1 small red onion sliced thin
1 small can of pitted whole black olives

Dressing:
1/4 cup of grated parmesan cheese
1 tblsp olive oil
¼ cup of balsamic vinegar

*toss all salad ingredients together in a oversized bowl
*combine all dressing ingredients in a small plastic bowl with a tight top and shake until blended
*immediately before serving, toss salad and dressing together

BodyInstinct Meatballs & Spaghetti Squash
1 pound of organic or steroid free lean ground beef (or turkey breast)
½ cup grated parmesan cheese
1 tbsp minced onion
½ cup Italian style Progresso Panko bread crumbs
1 teaspoon garlic salt
½ teaspoon pepper
1 egg
1 jar of prepared spaghetti sauce such as Paul Newman's
1 medium spaghetti squash

*mix all ingredients together except spaghetti squash
*make meatballs the size of golf balls and place in frying pan coated with cooking spray or olive oil
*brown on med high heat
*drain pain if necessary and add spaghetti sauce.
*simmer stirring often while you cook the squash
*deeply puncture squash several times with knife
*place in microwave oven and cook on high for 10 minutes
*let cool for at least 5 minutes then cut in half and scrape out seeds and center "gunk"
*scrape out squash onto plate (looks like yellow spaghetti) and add sauce and meatballs over top

BodyInstinct Corn Tortilla Quesadilla

2 small soft corn tortillas
3 oz can of chicken breast or 3 oz of fresh cooked chicken
½ cup of lowfat organic cheese shredded (mild cheddar or mozzarella or mix)
1 tbsp of refried beans with no lard
1 tblsp of all natural guacamole
1 tblsp of salsa

Spread beans on one tortilla
Mix chicken and cheese and spread on top of beans
Cover with other tortilla and grill in pan on medium until cheese is melted
Remove from grill and top with guacamole and salsa

BodyInstinct Baltimore Steamed Shrimp

1 pound of shrimp with shells on
¼ cup of Old Bay seasoning
¼ cup of coarse salt (kosher salt)

Place shrimp in a steamer that has come to a full boil.
Sprinkle Old Bay and salt on top of shrimp
Cover and steam for 2½ minutes
Uncover and stir shrimp
Replace cover and steam for 2½ more minutes
Immediately remove shrimp from pot and enjoy alone or with cocktail sauce
Served with a vegetable or salad

Gail's Stuffed Zucchini

3 med – large zucchini
1 lb. lean sausage (turkey, chicken, or pork) chopped up
½ cup Progresso Italian Style Panko Bread Crumbs
1 cup parmesan cheese

1 large clove of garlic minced
1 32 oz jar of spaghetti sauce
½ cup shredded part skim mozzarella (organic or Kraft hormone free)

Preheat oven to 350 degrees
Trim stems from the zucchini and slice lengthwise.
Scoop out the seeds, chop and put in bowl
Mix seeds with sausage, garlic, bread crumbs and parmesan cheese.
Stuff squash with sausage mixture and place in a 9x13 baking pan
Pour sauce over squash and cover pan with foil.
Bake for 45 minutes or until sausage is cooked.
Remove foil and sprinkle on mozzarella cheese.
Cook uncovered until cheese is melted.

BodyInstinct Corn and Bean Salsa
1 can black beans drained and rinsed
1 can corn drained
1 batch scallions chopped
1 yellow pepper chopped
4 oz lowfat feta cheese
¼ cup apple cider vinegar
¼ cup olive oil
1½ tsp sugar

Mix altogether and chill. May be served with baked corn chips or Tostito's scoops for a party dish or used as a topping for chicken or fish

BodyInstinct Fish Sticks
1½ pounds of white firm fish. (I have found Tilapia works best)
2 eggs beaten
1 cup of Progresso Italian Style Panko Bread Crumbs
1 cup grated parmesan cheese

*combine bread crumbs and parmesan
*cut fish into "sticks"
*dip fish sticks into beaten eggs and then into parmesan/bread crumb mixture
*put sticks on cookie sheet coated with cooking spray
*bake in 450 degree oven for 5 minutes
*take out pan and flip the sticks and bake another 5 minutes
*serves 4 or freeze some of the sticks for another meal!

ABOUT THE AUTHOR

A consummate health & fitness professional who doesn't just practice, but *lives* what she preaches, Tari inspires clients, readers and viewers with her knowledge and style.

When a paralyzing neurological and muscular illness, Guillian Barre' Syndrome abruptly ended her classical dance career, Tari learned the body's tenacity first-hand. After becoming completely paralyzed from the neck down followed by a year in physical therapy she developed a commitment to learning and understanding anatomy and physiology and started her new career in health & fitness, one that has flourished.

A sought-after Health & fitness lecturer, Tari delivers motivating and inspiring seminars and speeches on all aspects of health, fitness and nutrition. She has served as a speaker at both the **Disney Marathon**s and the **Disney Princess Marathons**.

As a free-lance writer, TV guest, motivational speaker and actress Tari has passionately shared her fitness philosophies and talents with many. She has been featured in health & fitness segments on major networks and has movie credits both in front of the camera and behind the scenes, preparing actors physically for their roles.

Most of her time is devoted to helping others who face challenges with their weight to overcome their real and perceived obstacles with the BodyInstinct Program. As a Mom she is also devoted to educating children about good nutrition and fitness.

www.TariRose.com

143

Made in the USA
Charleston, SC
23 January 2013